0

I dedicate this book to Helen Renée Wuorio.

My inspiration, and my reason.

# The
# 70 Second Difference™

**Politically Incorrect. Brutally Effective. Occasionally Amusing.**

**A Practical Guide to Exercise, Diet,**

**and Getting into Shape**

**Published by**

## MajorVision International

### 2016

Approved by The World Isometric Exercise Association

www.TWiEA.com

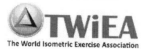

The World Isometric Exercise Association

Artwork and design: **WWW.MAJORVISION.COM**
WWW.MAJORVISION.COM

# Contents

*Important General Safety and Health Guidelines*

1. *Introduction*

2. *The Current Confusion*

3. *You Are What You Eat*

4. *Genetics, Epigenetics, and "Stuff"*

5. *Body Basics*

6. *The Science of Exercise*

7. *A Brief History of Isometric Exercise*

8. *Isometric Exercise Techniques*

9. *The 70 Second Difference™ Workout*

10. *Conclusion*

## *Important General Safety and Health Guidelines*

This section entitled, "Important General Safety and Health Guidelines," pertains to The ISOfitness™ Exercise System, and all books and publications about it not limited to but including The ISO90™ Course, Fitness on the Move™, The 70 Second Difference™, The Bullworker Bible™, the Sixty Second Ass Workout™, The Bullworker 90™ Course, The Bullworker Compendium™, Workout at Work™, The Doorway to Strength™, TRISOmetrics™, TRISOmetric™, the TRISOmetric™ system, ISOmetrics, The ISOmetric Bible™, the Iso-Bow® System, recommendations, suggestions, coaching, and advice, either written, verbal, in audio format, on video, written, or given, implied, or suggested the authors, from Brian Sterling-Vete, Helen Renée Wuorio, and the works thereof.

You should never begin any kind of sport, exercise system, workout plan, or diet modification, including everything contained in this book and in any books mentioned in the beginning paragraph above unless you have consulted with and have the full approval of your medical doctor.

Your physician can properly assess your current health status, and your ability to perform the exercises in the book and/or course. This is particularly important if you have any known or unknown pre-existing health issues, if you're pregnant, or if you believe that you may have other serious health conditions.

It's essential that you must always have the absolute approval from your physician before starting. Please show all the material in the above courses, books, video/audio, online material, and their content to your physician and get their approval before you start.

All exercises, suggestions, recommendations, instructions, exercise plans, dietary and eating recommendations, either given or implied, are intended only as a reference, and they are no substitute for a qualified professional personal coach who can help you to plan an exercise and diet program appropriate for your age and physical condition. Never overexert yourself when performing any exercise.

Stop exercising immediately and consult your doctor if you ever experience any pain, irregular heartbeat, shortness of breath, tightness in your chest/arms/fingers, faintness, nausea, or feelings of dizziness. Then consult your doctor and/or call the EMS immediately.

The exercises, courses, plans, and dietary recommendations in this book together with all those mentioned in all the books, general publications, online material, and videos mentioned in the names in paragraph 1 of this section, are not intended for use by children. Keep all exercise equipment out of the reach of children.

Always inspect any exercise equipment, and/or any/all other improvised or specifically made exercise equipment/materials, doors, door jambs, and door frames, and anything else you use before each use to ensure its proper operation and to ensure that it is undamaged and safe. Do not use it unless all parts are free from wear, and it is functioning properly. To avoid serious injury, care should always be taken using any/all exercise equipment, and in all items, people, books and courses, mentioned in paragraph 1 of this section.

Care should always be taken when getting into all exercise positions, on and off the floor, on and off chairs, on and off benches, on and off any other surface that might be used for exercise, including pieces of furniture, and in the use of all exercised equipment, either purpose made or improvised.

The creators, writers, instructors, originators, and owners of The Bullworker90™ Course, The ISO90 Course™, TRISOmetrics™, and all other courses, publications on video, audio, and in print, together with the courses, and websites, owned, originated, and created by the copyright holders and the ISOfitness™ team, including all books, courses, and people mentioned in paragraph 1 of this section, accept no responsibility whatsoever for any injury, harm, damage, illness, harm, damage to property, or any other negative health-related condition which may occur as a direct, or indirect result of following these courses, recommendations, suggestions, diagrams, pictures, videos, or while performing any exercises in these or any related other related material/publication/s.

For additional general information, we also recommend that you check reputable accredited medical advice sites, such as the two listed below.

The National Health Service in the United Kingdom, online at:
https://www.nhs.uk/Livewell/fitness/pages/physical-activity-guidelines-for-adults.aspx

In the USA, The Mayo Clinic online:
http://www.mayoclinic.org/healthy-lifestyle/fitness/in-depth/exercise/art-20047414

## Chapter 1: Introduction

All book titles and advertisement headlines are designed to catch the attention of potential customers. If this practice wasn't followed, then no matter how good the product was, no one would ever get to hear about it, or have the opportunity of becoming a new customer. The analogy would be of a guy winking at a pretty girl in the dark, no matter how hard he tried, he'd never stand a chance of getting a date because she'd never even know she was being winked at.

The title of this book is certainly no exception to that. However, if you're reading this far, then you've either expressed a strong enough interest to electronically "thumb" a few pages to browse the content on Amazon, or you've already bought it. If the latter is the case, then thank you, and we sincerely hope that you enjoy this book. Either way, the point I'm making is that your interest will have been aroused. You will have been attracted to the book because of certain drivers, desires and needs, combined with curiosity about what you've read so far.

We're completely transparent in our belief that people who read this book will either love it, or hate it, and there will be very few who fall into a grey area of middle ground. This is because we're not just another book which conforms to the accepted cosy beliefs most people have about diet and exercise. Far from it. We're the people who tend to be branded as "controversial," because we will set aside any preconceived thoughts and accepted beliefs to look at a subject with an open mind. For most closed-minded people, the subject of diet/nutrition and exercise, and their beliefs which surround it is almost like a religion. They simply cannot and will not accept even the possibility of there being an alternative way. In their mind, it is all "set in stone." Even though they purport to others that they follow proven science, few, if any, will dare to think that their "accepted" beliefs about the subject might be flawed in some way.

Whoever you are, and whatever you might have thought and believed about the subject of diet/nutrition and exercise until now, we can only ask that when you read this book you will at least try to keep an open mind about the subject. My partner and I have practised and researched these subjects for a total of almost 60 years, both formally at university, and as our life-passion. During this time, we have discovered many new things, some of which might be life-changing to many, and this is part of our way of sharing our discoveries with the world.

### The Obligatory "Stuff" About Us

To begin this obligatory, and self-serving section, I'd like to begin by introducing my partner and co-author, Helen Renée Wuorio.

I first met Helen when she was training for a Bikini Fitness competition in 2015, and she initially caught my attention because of the dramatic transformation she'd achieved in a short period of time. I also took notice of her because I was struck by her open-minded thirst for knowledge about the most effective, and efficient, ways to exercise.

I was particularly impressed by the fact that despite

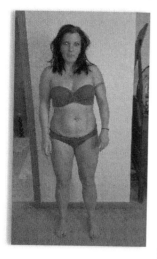

her many years spent eating an appallingly unhealthy diet, together with overcoming many other personal challenges, how, in only 8 months of training, Helen had managed to transform her body from being 40lbs overweight, to become a Bikini Fitness Bodybuilding competitor. More importantly, Helen had used what I considered to be outmoded, traditional exercise methods, together with a flawed diet, and she'd managed to place 2$^{nd}$ and 4$^{th}$ place respectively, in her first Bikini Fitness competition.

Perhaps it is the adversities we all face in life that become the primary motivators which ultimately drive us on to our personal successes. Overcoming common adversities in life allow us to more effectively relate and empathise with others who also want to make changes, but don't know where to start, and

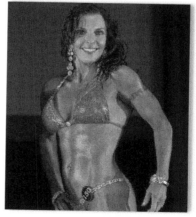

what to do next. Many of the challenges and adversities which Helen has battled, and then overcome, have been the same as those which we all face in life. Therefore, Helen can relate directly to the clients and customers of both sexes who reach out to her, and who need help with their own similar issues.

Helen has a refreshing, new-found dedication and approach to pursuing only the most efficient forms of exercise and the healthiest nutrition systems. She is passionate about exercise science, and how it can be translated into practical exercise methods that can be easily practised and followed by most people.

Now that I've introduced Helen, I'll now write a little bit about myself. I'm told I'm supposed to do this because it will make me appear to be more important than I am. I also take complete responsibility for every ounce of irony in those last lines. The bottom line is that this section is supposed to validate why you have spent money on this book, instead of spending it on going out for a good time with your friends. Therefore, I hope that it does the trick.

Perhaps it's not quite as brutal as that. However, you're probably wondering who I am, what my background

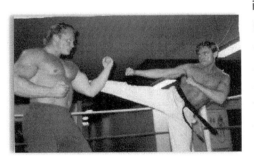 is, and why I believe that I'm qualified to write a book about exercise. Therefore, here's the "obligatory" part about me.

I've led what can be termed as being a "colourful life," which really means that it's been somewhat varied, and not what might be called "typical." This is because I've

been told by many that it's not especially "typical" to have been part of the team who were the main sponsors of the Tyrrell Formula 1 racing team or to have spent over a decade travelling around the world with BBC News. Apparently, it's not "typical" to have once held 5 World records, with my last Guinness World Record still standing at the time of writing.

Now we've established that my life to date hasn't been "typical," I'll tell you more about my experience in exercise science. I've spent nearly 5 decades researching and studying all forms of exercise, fitness, strength, and general resistance training. During that time, I've been both a professional athlete and a professional coach. Since the time when I first began exercising, I've tried and tested almost every kind of exercise concept, exercise equipment, training course, and diet plan that was invented or devised. In addition, I've lifted hundreds of tons in weight over the years during my exercise sessions. This is because exercise, fitness, strength training, and a healthy diet have been an integral part of my entire life.

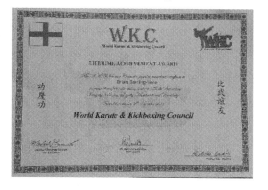

I've practised the martial arts regularly since I was 12 years old. The result of almost 50 years of practice has been my receiving 4 black belts, a lifetime achievement award, and being appointed as "World Coach" by the World Karate and Kickboxing Council. I formally studied the subject of sports science at university, I competed as an amateur in all-natural (no-steroid) bodybuilding competitions, in highland games, strength events, and in competitive martial arts. Eventually, I became a full-time professional in a combination of these two disciplines.

I've owned, and at times co-owned, several commercial fitness studios and gyms, I've devised major new ranges of bodybuilding and sports nutrition supplements for large corporations, I've worked alongside British Olympic Games coaches, I've designed gym equipment for major manufacturers, and I provided the technical consultancy needed to design major fitness centres such as the one at H.M.S. Excellent in Portsmouth, England, for the Royal Navy and the Royal Marines Commandos.

I was a coach to my friend, the great Jon Pall Sigmarsson of Iceland, who was 4 times World's Strongest Man. At the time of writing, I believe that Jon Pall still holds the world record for deadlifting half a ton. This was a 1,253lb lift, in competition against two other mighty opponents and multi World's

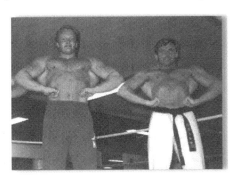

*Brian and 4 Time World's Strongest Man: Jon Pall Sigmarsson*

Strongest Man winners, Geoff Capes and Bill Kazmaier.

When I expanded my business interests into the world of television, I naturally began producing videos

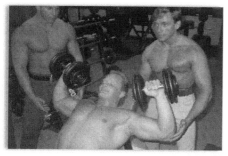

about exercise, sports science, athletic performance, and weight training. Many of these were sold via the UK's National Coaching Foundation, and the YMCA.

In 2015, a major US-based publishing company even rated me as being one of the top fitness coaches in America. Maybe I am, or maybe I'm not, I don't really know the answer to that, because it's all very subjective. Furthermore, I've absolutely no idea how they reached that conclusion, and it was very nice to receive such a wonderful compliment. It's been accepted graciously, in the spirit in which it was given.

This has been a brief overview of my exercise-related life to date. However, since I first began STUDYING exercise science at university in the late 1970s, I've amassed a huge library of research notes, data, rare journals, and other material about the science of exercise. In fact, a lot of the scientific data in this book is taken from that library, and from my PhD research notes.

Therefore, in terms of exercise, I've seen a lot, I've done a lot, I've experienced a lot, and I've learned a lot along the way. In fact, I'd even go so far as to say that I've probably forgotten more than many of the "new-kid-on-the-block" coaches have learned to date.

I may not sound very modest in saying that I'm a good exercise coach, but that is exactly what I believe to be true. Perhaps the proverbial "proof of the pudding" in this respect is in the national, international, and World Champions I've helped to coach successfully over 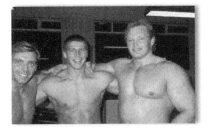 the years because they're the real testimony to what I know about the subject.

To summarise this obligatory, and self-promoting section, all this information tells you that I've got slightly more than an average knowledge of the subject of exercise, fitness, strength training, body shaping, and bodybuilding. Since this is the case, my advice might be worth taking in this respect. At the very least, my thoughts about exercise science might be worth considering. I'll stop now, especially since I've probably bored you to the point of proverbially "gnawing your paw off" to try and escape this section.

## Choosing a Good Coach

No book, course, website or magazine is ever going to be as good as having an experienced, and knowledgeable coach. One-to-one coaching is always going to be the best, and everything else is an acceptable substitute.

However, during my travels around the world, and especially around the USA, I've met and encountered many coaches. Some of them were excellent, with some even being outstanding in their field. Unfortunately, many others were woefully ignorant of even basic exercise science. In fact, I've met some "coaches" who I believe would find it challenging if they were ever competing on a TV general knowledge quiz show against an opponent that was nothing more than an average potato bought from a supermarket.

From the way some of the new "whizz-kid-coaches" talk, you'd think they had invented the subject of exercise, and that they absolutely "knew it all." Of course, the reality is that they didn't invent the subject.

However, some of them seem to have convinced themselves that they did. What's more, despite what they want to believe, they certainly don't know everything about exercise. FAR from it in fact. No one can know "everything" about exercise because we're all still learning and new discoveries are being made every day.

The problem for the average customer is in choosing a good one. If you visit the average gym, you can easily spot many coaches who simply hang around, hoping to pick up a new client either by luck or via a recommendation of some sort. The problem for the customer is that most of these coaches have only completed a short online course in exercise and coaching. They've never studied the subject for years academically, and they've completed their online course by taking mostly "true or false" or multiple-choice exams.

Once this is over, if they've reached a high enough average score, then BINGO, they're suddenly a "fully qualified" coach! In the larger fitness clubs and national chains, they've even devised their own coaching courses and qualifications. Some of which are good, while others are not so good because there are no internationally recognised standards to adhere to.

*"I have an example of the coaches you can find today. I recently heard a coach announce dramatically online that oatmeal is bad for you.*

*I was curious about this because I had never heard that before, therefore, I wanted to hear the science and research behind this coach's reasoning as to why one should not eat oatmeal.*

*I listened intently to the online video blog as they rambled-on with nonsense about the donuts and other junk food they had eaten that day until finally, the coach says: "This is why you should not eat oatmeal... because it's gross!"*

*They then went on to say that it's also disgusting, and they don't know why anyone would ever eat it. I was in utter shock over this statement. Where was the science? Where is the research? There was none whatsoever!"*

When Helen told me about this "coach," I simply shook my head in disbelief. Seriously, I thought to myself? However, what scared me even more than what was said, was that this person apparently has a coaching qualification which allows them to teach exercise to poor, unsuspecting schmucks who genuinely want to get into shape. More importantly, these are the same coaching qualifications that are deemed to be "acceptable," and allow them to work in gyms and fitness clubs to teach exercise.

In my opinion, this sort of coaching certificate isn't even worth the paper it's printed on. They may as well be offered as a giveaway promotion with breakfast cereal. I can even imagine the advertisement for it. "Collect 'X' number of cereal packet coupons and become a fully qualified exercise coach!" It's scary stuff, and it's happening all around you now.

Don't get me wrong. There are many EXCELLENT coaches who are smart, and extremely knowledgeable. These coaches aren't hard to find either, you just need to do a little research, and not be afraid to ask a few direct questions about who they are,

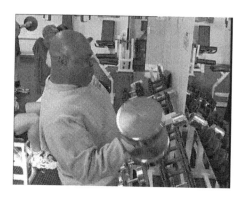

*Powerlifiting Strength Phenomenon: 'Big' Ricky Richardson*

what they're qualified to teach, and how they received their qualification.

I've had the privilege to either know and/or to work with some of the finest coaches in the world. People like 2 times World's Strongest Man winner Geoff Capes, and Pure Strength winner Hjalti Árnason, together with coaches like: Jamie Baird, John Cupello, Tommy Wood, 'Big' Ricky

Richardson, John Carrigan, John Robertson, and of course 3-time World Muay Thai Champion, 2-time World Martial Arts Champion, and The King of Thailand's Champion: the great Stuart Hurst.

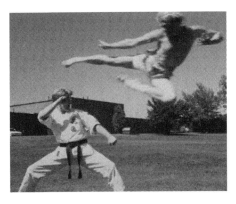

*3-Time World Muay Thai Champion and 2-Time World Martial Arts Champion: Stuart Hurst*

These people are all outstanding coaches and specialists in their field. Both Helen and I are proud to know them. Therefore, when you're searching for a coach, we strongly urge you to do plenty of research and don't be afraid to ditch them fast, if they ever devise plans for you which make no scientific sense.

## What is ISOfitness™?

The ISOfitness™ exercise system is the name we use to cover all the applied exercises we have devised especially for the ISOfitness™ exercise system and which we write about and teach. All exercises in the ISOfitness™ system should be performed in specific ways and combinations, and include isometric, isokinetic, and combined isotonic exercises. The core of the ISOfitness™ exercise system is based solidly on the original proven isometric science and was developed from there. However, the ISOfitness™ system is much more than that alone. It incorporates the

23

new and advanced isometric exercise discoveries with techniques including, Dynamic Flexation™, Super-Slow Isotonic Flexation™, and the newly proven science of USB-UHT™ (Ultra Short Burst – Ultra High Intensity) exercises. The ISOFitness™ exercise system also includes our own resultant hybrid TRISOmetric™ exercise system.

## *TWiEA™ Resources.*

All ISOfitness™ online resources have now been absorbed into The World Isometric Exercise Association, or TWiEA™ for short (www.TWiEA.com). The World Isometric Exercise Association, TWiEA™, is the global governing body for all types of isometric exercise. TWiEA™'s mission is to help set and maintain standards of excellence in teaching and promoting all types of isometric exercise

It was formed because most exercise coaches and gyms don't promote and recommend isometric exercises is because of the following: A) they lack the required training/real knowledge to teach isometrics properly, B) they have self-serving commercial interests which mean that recommending isometric exercise could deeply impact their training/membership fees.

it's ironic that the exercise systems that most exercise professionals recommend to their clients are the systems that take the most time to perform. Therefore, they're the exercise systems that people will most likely stop using! In the global quest to improve health and fitness by encouraging people to exercise regularly using traditional time-consuming methods, coaches and personal trainers who do this are actually compounding matters to become part of the overall problem. Since lack of time is typically the #1 reason restricting and/or preventing people from getting the high-level workout they need, coaches should be recommending real-life time-efficient exercise solutions that busy people can follow.

TWiEA™'s mission is to ensure that scientifically proven time-efficient isometric exercise techniques are taught to clients as part of an integrated overall approach to the total-body exercise solutions provided by fitness professionals. This creates a much higher probability that clients who are busy people, and who often face real-life time-crunches, can still maintain a regular highly effective exercise program.

The fact is that isometric exercise is every bit as effective, and frequently more effective, at building muscle and strength as other more traditional forms of resistance training. It is also a time-saving and money-saving exercise solution that almost anyone can perform, even without equipment.

## *What is "The 70 Second Difference™?"*

"The 70 Second Difference™" is a new approach to exercise which focusses on the scientifically proven superior isometric exercise system, together with the proven benefits of extremely short, yet high-intensity isotonic exercise sessions. It also incorporates functional Isokinetic, and adaptive response™ exercise. We use the term "functional Isokinetic" in respect of how these exercises can be performed in practical ways by employing self-resisted force, with a constant velocity.

25

"The 70 Second Difference™" is also about time. Lack of time is the traditional enemy of strength, fitness, and bodybuilding, and to a degree, we've all been conditioned over the years to subconsciously believe that a workout session will take between 30 and 60 minutes to perform. Indeed, lack of time is widely recognised as being the number one reason why people either don't exercise or why they stop exercising.

Even the most dedicated exercise enthusiast who has relatively easy access to traditional exercise equipment will sooner or later be forced to skip workouts due to lack of time. The inevitable time-crunches of life, family, and work are something that we all face, and with seemingly increasing regularity when the demands of work are particularly intense.

This is hardly surprising, especially when one considers how long it takes to attend a traditional gym or fitness club to maintain a regular workout schedule. Being a member of a gym can be incredibly time-consuming. In just one week, someone who exercises regularly, 3 evenings each week, can easily spend the equivalent of a full working day doing that. Even if the average workout or exercise class can be completed in 60 minutes, the travel time there and back, traffic delays, parking hassles, changing and shower room time, searching for a vacant locker, and waiting for equipment at peak times etc. can make a single gym visit a 3-hour ordeal. Even traditional home exercise systems still require a significant time-commitment for them to be effective and deliver the desired results. Even "convenient" traditional home gym systems will still usually require between 20 and 60 minutes of exercise time to complete a workout.

"The 70 Second Difference™" concept follows the science. Independent scientific research has proven beyond doubt that extremely intense exercise that is performed for only very brief periods, lasting no more than several seconds, can be of equal, or often greater benefit to as much as an hour of traditional lower intensity exercise. Science has also proven the superiority of isometric exercise, and since these exercises only take between 7 and 10 seconds to perform, therefore, it is an ideal combination.

"The 70 Second Difference™" workout involves performing only 7 high-intensity exercises, performed over 70 seconds of consecutive exercise time, and only once each day. These exercises have been carefully designed to exercise all the major muscle groups of the body, while at the same time stimulating your Base Metabolic Rate (BMR), 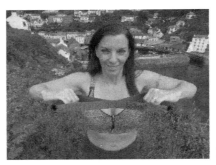 increase your functional strength, sculpt your muscles, and increase your overall fitness level. These exercises are based on the proven science of maximum efficiency ISOfitness™ system. This makes it is almost impossible *not* to be able find the time you need to exercise, even on your busiest day.

It's just a fact that everyone, no matter how busy they are, can always find 70 seconds of spare time in any given day.  This means that you always have time to perform "The 70 Second Difference™" workout, even on the busiest of days.  If you believe that you can't spare just 70 seconds out of the 86,400 seconds in your day, then you're just making sad excuses why you *can't* exercise, instead of finding good reasons why you can.  The person who makes that decision is you.

When we devised "The 70 Second Difference™" concept, we took the 7 basic exercises that can be performed with an Iso-Bow®, or a pair of Iso-Bows®, which exercise all the main muscle groups to give a total-body workout.  These exercises can be performed in what we call an almost zero-footprint workout environment.  This means that you can perform them almost anywhere.  in the time it's taken us to write our books, and while filming our exercise videos, we've travelled extensively.  However, we've always used the "The 70 Second Difference™" exercise system, so we've never missed a workout.  We've had a total-body workout on a plane trip, as a passenger in a car, and on train journeys too.  You never have to miss a workout ever again, it doesn't matter if you're travelling away from home on business, on holiday, or if for some reason you find yourself in a remote and exotic location.

"The 70 Second Difference™" concept and the ISOfitness™ exercise system is deceptively powerful.  They can be used with equal effectiveness by people of all levels of strength and fitness because they harness the body's natural Adaptive Response mechanism.  The Adaptive Response mechanism is how your body naturally adjusts to force and intensity it applies to all self-resisted isometric and isotonic exercises.  The harder, and more intensity you apply with one body part or muscle group, the greater the counter-resistance generated from the opposing counterparts. The Adaptive Response mechanism also means that a person who is already strong and fit, can naturally apply much greater force and intensity to an exercise than a weaker, less fit person. However, if for example, both people apply 2/3rds of their overall personal maximum strength, they will both still receive approximately the same percentage of benefit in return.

Therefore, it doesn't matter how big or strong you are, to begin with, you will still be challenged if you genuinely apply the appropriate level of force and intensity to any of the exercises in "The 70 Second Difference™" exercise concept. If you're a complete beginner, perhaps even someone who has never exercised before, then by applying the same principles, you will receive similar benefits in return. The harder you work, the greater the results, and the faster they will be delivered.

We're confident that anyone who tries "The 70 Second Difference™" workout and applies the appropriate levels of force and intensity according to their abilities, they will be able to feel the results from their very first workout, and within 5 days they'll begin to see results too.

## Chapter 2: The Current Confusion

Today, for people who know little or nothing about exercise and diet, the subject is more confusing than ever before. There are a plethora of choices all wrapped-up in marketing hype. There are more gadget exercise devices than ever before on the market, all manner of diets and eating plans, and for the layperson, it's tough to even come close to making the right choice about what works, and what doesn't.

For example, there are a vast number of cleverly named diet systems and eating plans made to sound like

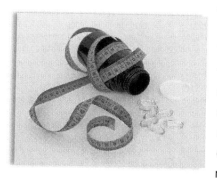

they're "medical" or "genetic" in some way. These pathetically transparent systems are either ordinarily sensible eating plans sold under a fancy name and price, or they're ineffective rubbish. They're often nothing more than a basic vitamin supplement of some sort, packaged in marketing hype to sell for extortionate prices to people who simply don't know any better. Some products even directly insult people. They suggest that their customers who want to lose weight, somehow can't make the direct connection that eating less generally leads to weight loss. Obviously, the subject of weight loss can be more complex at times. However, in and of itself, in respect of weight loss, there is always going to be a direct connection between the amount of food consumed, and the weight of the individual. It's not a rocket science connection. Most of these supplements aren't necessary, people simply need to make better daily food choices and take a little exercise.

Even though most of the home exercise gadgets are typically useless, people still fall for the same ridiculous sales hype of alluring infomercials and adverts. At best, some of the machines and gadgets we've seen recently might provide a reasonably good workout, however, this is usually only delivered to comparatively small areas of the body. The higher quality devices, such as commercial grade treadmills and stepper combinations, carry a very hefty price tag, and 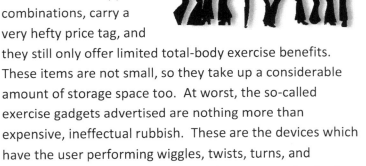 they still only offer limited total-body exercise benefits. These items are not small, so they take up a considerable amount of storage space too. At worst, the so-called exercise gadgets advertised are nothing more than expensive, ineffectual rubbish. These are the devices which have the user performing wiggles, twists, turns, and wobbles, of various kinds. They might appear to be fun in the TV commercial, however, they don't really do very much in terms of body shaping, weight loss, and increasing strength.

There are some exercise systems and routines advertised which do nothing more than "wiggle your arse" dance classes sold on DVD. It should be blatantly obvious to a blind person on a very dark night that they're being asked to pay a lot of money for a few dance class videos packaged as a "state of the art" exercise system. I'm sure that most people reading this now will have seen these commercials. The elaborate dance parties performed by well-choreographed professional dancers, who are already in great shape, and with the voice-over saying something like "Shipped to your door on DVD for only 3 easy payments of X, plus postage and packing." Unfortunately, the producers of these systems target the vulnerable people who have no knowledge about exercise. The people who cling on to the belief that somehow by having fun, and waggling their wobbly bits to music, is going to be all that's needed for them to be miraculously transformed. Somehow, after completing the course, they'll look more like the models and athletes who perform the dance routines in the multi DVD boxed sets.

Admittedly, these dance routines will certainly help to increase a person's cardiovascular efficiently and burn some calories in the process, but at what cost? Exercise systems such as these usually cost somewhere between $50 and $100, which is a lot of money. The same results could be easily achieved at zero expense, by simply dancing around the lounge while listening to music on any CD or DVD. At least a person's own CD or DVD collection would contain their favourite tracks, which are always going to be much better than license-fee "rubbishmusic.com" stuff which is often used in commercial dance-exercise DVD's.

It's a similar story when it comes to infomercials selling expensive exercise systems which are really nothing more than regular HIIT, or High-Intensity Interval Training routines. Again, these routines are nicely packaged and wrapped in marketing hype, complete with a catchy name. Naturally, paying a lot of money for what is nothing more than a cleverly packaged regular HIIT system is well worth it, especially since you may win a cheap t-shirt at the end of it all. Right? We're not saying that these expensive commercially packaged HIIT workout systems won't deliver some good results, because when used properly, they will. They'll get you really fit, they'll burn calories, increase your BMR, they'll provide great overall health benefits. When used in combination with a good eating plan, then the user will probably lose weight too. However, the point that we're making here is that you don't need to spend a lot of money to achieve the same results, all it takes is a little independent thought and willpower.

On a slightly different note, we never cease to be amazed at the advertisements and infomercials for exercise gadgets that advertise the "regular value" of the product is much more than what's being asked during the commercial. Not to mention the "but wait! We'll ship you two for the price of one if you buy within the next 60 seconds!" Hello? This commercial hype is completely insulting to all intelligent viewers. People simply need to do a little research into what they really need to exercise inexpensively, and efficiently. However, for many people, and especially for those who usually tend to shop late at night, it somehow seems to make perfect sense to buy-into the easy, fun-based solution they see in the infomercial.

Here's the bad news. The advertisers and manufacturers of these products don't really care if what they're selling works, or not. By the time the buyer has discovered that the overpriced plastic gadget doesn't work, it's too late. The people selling it already have the money so they don't really care.

The viewing public seems to be split into two groups. One group consists of intelligent people who think for themselves. People with an open mind, who are prepared to really work at something, and who are interested in getting good value combined with real results. The other group seems to consist of people who will continue to waste money in the vain hope that eventually one of the "effortless" exercise gadgets might work. The sort of people who are seeking what we call the "Cinderella exercise effect." The problem is that they've got more chance of waiting for their personal "fairy godmother" to materialise before their eyes, and then wave a transformation magic wand at them.

Are there some people who are really that stupid? Yes, it seems that there really are a lot of stupid people in the world. After all, if there weren't customers for these things, then there wouldn't be the huge quantity of rubbish exercise gadgets marketed via ridiculous infomercials would there?

We're certain that everyone reading these words right now, have at some point encountered, and been frustrated by stupid people. Therefore, we thought that you might be really interested to find out that the "stupid people phenomena" has even been scientifically proven to exist. The subject of "stupid people" was officially researched in a series of experiments performed by David Dunning and Justin Kruger in the department of psychology at Cornell University, in the USA. Unsurprisingly, the phenomenon is called "The Dunning-Kruger Effect" and you can get more data about it at the following websites: http://www.livescience.com/18678-incompetent-people-

ignorant.html and
https://en.wikipedia.org/wiki/Dunning%E2%80%93Kruger_
effect

Now that we've made a somewhat sarcastic, and cutting, appraisal of some of the choices people are faced with when it comes to buying exercise courses and fitness equipment, what about ISOfitness™ and "The 70 Second Difference™" concept? Where does that fit into the "useless to excellent" scale of things? Naturally, we think that our concepts sit high, towards the "excellent" end of the scale, and only modesty prevents us from saying that they're the very best. We believe in our system because independent science has proven that it works very effectively. The tests to determine this have been performed by some of the world's leading sports scientists and physiologists, at some of the finest research establishments and universities in the world. Therefore, we can categorically state that the science behind the workout routines and exercises in the ISOfitness™ system, and in this book, all have the following things in common:

- They Really Work.
- They're Easy to Learn.
- They Take Very Little Time to Perform.
- Almost Anyone Can Do Them.
- It's an Inexpensive, Yet Highly Effective Exercise System.

Not many, if any, of the infomercial advertised systems, can honestly say the same thing. Especially since many make wild claims about their products based solely on their own self-commissioned "research."

## Responsibility Today

Today, more than ever before, people seem to have an increasing problem in taking responsibility for their own actions. You've only got to look at people at your work, and in your social life, to see what we mean in this respect.

Many people, and especially some of the young people in society today, believe that they aren't responsible for anything in life. They have a disgustingly huge, and unrealistic sense of entitlement, and a completely unrealistic expectation about what life is all about.

The real problems begin, especially for everyone on the "fallout" zone around them when people like this are forced to face up to life and harsh reality. When they collide with the immovable object known as reality, many of them have what can only be described as a "tantrum" moment. To take responsibility for your own actions should be a given. However, for many people today it's all about how they can avoid being responsible for as much as possible, and how they can blame someone else for everything they can possibly get away with.

Certain pathetic members of the legal profession have helped to turn the art of "not taking responsibility for one's own actions" into a growing cancer which is helping to ruin western society. The members of the legal profession who do this may gain a little financially every time they win a ridiculous lawsuit which supports an individual's stupidity, however, it's always going to be a hollow and shameful victory that causes the sane and sensible members of the public to grow to increasingly despise them.

In terms of exercise, fitness, weight loss, and body shape, the problem of people not wanting to take responsibility for themselves is a huge issue. More importantly, it's an issue that society can no longer afford to ignore or pretend that it doesn't exist.

## Plexcuses

In life, there will always be plenty of people who seem to specialise in making excuses for why they can't do something. It doesn't matter what it is, they're simply negative about everything. This is especially true about why they can't seem to get themselves into good physical condition. These people are experts in this highly questionable art form, and they create some amazing almost completely plausible excuses. We call these almost logical, and seemingly plausible excuses: "plexcuses." Plexcuses are the sorts of excuses, which, seem to make enough sense so that the listener doesn't stop to think too deeply about what's just been said. Therefore, they tend to automatically accept what they're being told.

If you're one of these people, then, after reading this book and facing a few indisputable facts, if you continue to try and dream up more plexcuses, they'll be so obviously transparent and thin, that they'll be positively anorexic in nature. You should be too embarrassed to even think about continuing to make those same old plexcuses.

Naturally, there are some people who have completely valid excuses about why they have serious issues with excess body weight. These people have genuine medical conditions. However, these conditions are usually extremely rare. Unfortunately, it's quite common to find that many people who have these issues, have self-created them. Typically, they've done this through making bad food choices, and a failure to exercise enough willpower.

When I was the owner of a small chain of fitness clubs, I had many direct experiences with clients who deliberately chose to use imaginary clinical health issues as their excuse for being overweight. In addition to this, many of these people had developed several psychosomatic symptoms of those medical conditions. One of the people I'm thinking about now as I write these words seemed to almost enjoy the attention it attracted because of it. I believe that the people who use these sorts of plexcuses are nothing more than bone-idle, weak-willed, and lazy. They simply lack the willpower, courage, and determination needed to get off their lazy backside and do something positive about their health.

---

### HELEN WRITES

**Helen Renée – The Former "Queen" of Plexcuses**

---

*I admit that I was once one of the excuse-driven people we write about, in fact at times I could have easily won a contest to become the "Queen of Plexcuses."*

*Since I was a teenager I've always struggled with my weight, and even though I was a gymnast and reasonably fit, there was always a little "belly pouch" which simply wouldn't go away. It never dawned on me that the processed breadsticks and the other junk food I was eating for lunch each day had anything to do with my extra belly fat. Thinking back, I now wonder how much better I'd have been at gymnastics if I'd only paid more attention to what I was eating. Throughout my 20's and 30's, I would continuously fluctuate between 10 and 30lbs overweight. I'd often try the latest diet trend, and the latest workout trend as well, which included Jazzercise, Pilates, and aerobics, etc. No matter what I did, I always chalked up my extra belly fat to my favourite "plexcuse," which was: "It's in my genetics." After all, most of the women in my family had the classic belly bulge.*

*In addition to this, once you've given birth to children, you have a plethora of new "plexcuses" to use. From that point onward, I could always blame my extra belly bulge on having two C-sections, in wanting to believe that I had no time to work-out, that the kids were sick, or that the kids had additional after-school activities. You name the "plexcuses," and I guarantee that I used it!*

*As the years passed, I approached my late 30's and eventually the dreaded 40-year milestone, only to find that I'd gained even more weight than ever. So, in my quest to counteract this flabby onslaught, I decided to train for a half-marathon. I joined a gym, I was on a strict 1400 calories a day diet, but at that point, I was doing mostly cardio exercises and minimal weight training. The result of all this was that I lost weight, and for the first time in 30 years, I achieved my target weight!*

*On my 40th birthday I completed my first half-marathon in 2 hours and 3 minutes, but annoyingly I still had a little belly bulge. What did I tell myself and others* about this? Of course, I reverted to it being the "it's in my genes" "plexcuse." Unfortunately, once the half-marathon was over and I cut back on my training, I quickly gained the weight back. However, over the next couple of years, I still completed a few more half-marathons, 5k's, and even 10k's, but no matter what I did, I still never got back to my original target weight. The simple fact was that I'd put the effort into training for running, but I hadn't been following any sort of reasonable diet.

Fast-forward to my mid 40's, and by that time I'm facing a 2nd divorce. As you might imagine, this wasn't exactly a "fun-filled" time in my life, and somehow, I felt like I'd once again failed both my family and myself. Over the following 10 months my body weight "ballooned" to the heaviest that I'd ever been in my life. The only saving grace was that being in the fashion industry I was always able to dress well, and cleverly hide the excess weight I was carrying.

At first glance to the untrained eye, no one could tell just how unfit I was, however, I felt it. I had a hard time

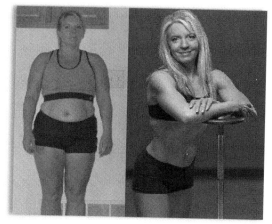

climbing stairs, walking long distances, and I completely lacked both energy and enthusiasm, which meant that I just wanted to sleep all the

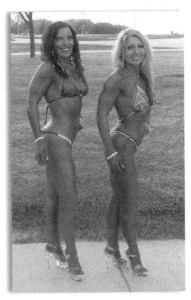

time. By this time, my twin sister, Rhonda, had also gained weight to the point where she'd become 50+lbs overweight, so she made a life-change. She hired a coach and announced to the family that she would be entering a bodybuilding competition to compete in the Figure Class.

I was extremely proud of her wanting to lose excess weight and build some muscle, however, I also hate to admit that I was completely sceptical about her ever achieving her target weight, and to be able to compete on stage in a bikini.

Even though part of me was sure that if she put the effort in, then she would eventually lose weight, I also thought to myself, "doesn't she realize the women in our family will never lose the belly?" After about 10 months of her training with weights, and following a strict diet, I was completely shocked to find that she'd done the unthinkable and she'd finally lost the belly! She looked incredible, and I could hardly believe my eyes. It was at that point when I realized something profound. I realised that anybody can

41

get into shape IF they want it bad enough and are determined enough. You must commit the time, effort, and research needed if you really want to succeed.

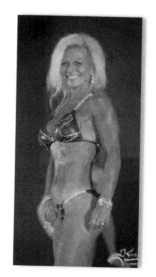

It was because of her amazing transformation that I then became inspired hire a coach and enter my first Bodybuilding Competition, in the Bikini Fitness Class. My best friend, Glenda Ama and I, decided to compete together. We agreed that we were ultimately responsible for the size and shape of our own bodies, and we made a pact to keep each other accountable if we strayed off-plan.

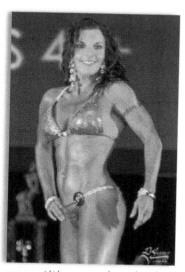

To compete, I needed to drop 40 lbs of excess fat, and she needed to drop 60 lbs, but the inspiration my twin sister had provided made us sure that we could do this! In only 8 months, we'd done it! We'd both made our target body weight, and our target body-fat percentages. That year we competed in our first competitions, and we both walked away with some trophies. I'd achieved that which I thought once was

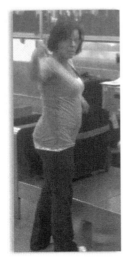

*impossible, I'd dropped 40lbs of excess fat, competed on stage in a bikini, and in the process, I'd earned a $2^{nd}$, $3^{rd}$ and a $4^{th}$ place in the competitions I entered that year.*

*That was the turning point in my life, and I had finally realised that I had made so many "plexcuses" over the years that it was positively*

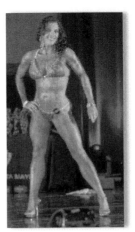

*embarrassing. I'd literally transformed myself in every way. If I'd have done this sooner, then I could have led a much healthier, fitter life in my 20's and 30's. From that point onward: NO MORE PLEXCUSES!*

## Political Correctness

As you may have gathered from the title of this book, we're not especially politically correct in our approach. Furthermore, We're proud of that. It's our

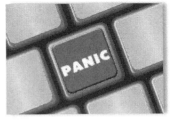

belief that political correctness isn't just counterproductive, it typically flies directly in the face of common sense. It usually makes little, or no, sense, and it has spread out like a contaminant across society.

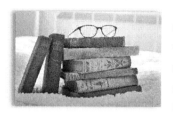

Since we're blunt in our approach and our choice of words, if you're easily offended, easily shocked, easily upset, easily appalled, then you might want to do the following: **STOP READING THIS BOOK RIGHT NOW.** Instead, find a book and exercise system that has a "bedside manner," which is more in keeping with what you're looking for. If you carry on reading from this point onward, then it's entirely your own choice. You have been clearly warned both on the book cover, and here as well. Our blunt approach might even make you stop and think laterally, independently, and more clearly about what really works and what doesn't when it comes to changing the size and shape of your body through diet and exercise.

If you do read on from this point, and then you suddenly decide that you're offended, you need to remember that **NOBODY FORCED YOU TO READ THIS BOOK, IT WAS YOUR DELIBERATE CHOICE TO DO THAT.** You didn't just happen to buy this book by accident, and then also read it by way of another accident.

We'd also like to clearly point out that we're not deliberately picking on anyone who is overweight or obese. We're not what's commonly known as "fattist," because we believe in freedom of choice. Therefore, if some people are genuinely happy being overweight and obese, that's great, good for them.

We're certainly not being deliberately anti-fat, far from it in fact. Everyone's decided weight, and body shape is always going to be a matter of personal choice. We wish

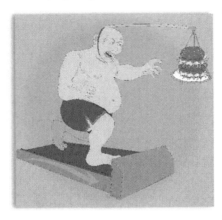

every person genuine happiness with their chosen individual body size, weight, and shape.

However, we're targeting our exercise system and approach to nutrition to people who may **also** include those who are overweight and obese, and who are seeking a no-nonsense approach to getting into shape and losing weight.

There are many coaches, authors, and websites that offer their clients and readers a much more sympathetic approach to becoming fitter and getting into shape. That's great, and we applaud them for taking that approach if that's what they think is best. If our approach isn't to your liking, then our advice is to find an approach that is.

If you're looking for what we call the "tea and sympathy" approach, then instead of reading this book and following our system, go and chat with your Mother, your best friend, or your significant other. They may even enjoy listening to you moan and complain about the size and shape of your body, and about how you struggle to eat less, and about your excuses as to why you don't exercise.

For far too long people have been coddled and fed with "fluffy," emotionally in-touch efforts to help them relate to how they can lose weight and get into shape. This "warm and fuzzy" bedside manner approach has obviously worked **REALLY** well. Yes, in case you were wondering, that last line was loaded with maximum sarcasm. To see exactly how the "fluffy," emotionally in-touch approach has failed miserably, you've only got to look around the average shopping mall, or a large public gathering to see how there are more people than ever before who are hugely obese. The official statistics published on the United States Center for Disease Control and Prevention website (source: http://www.cdc.gov/nchs/fastats/obesity-overweight.htm) are nothing short of alarming. They are as follows:

- △ Percentage of adults age 20 years and over with obesity: 37.9% (2013-2014)
- △ Percentage of adults age 20 years and over with overweight, including obesity: 70.7% (2013-2014)
- △ Percentage of adolescents age 12-19 years with obesity: 20.5% (2011-2012)
- △ Percentage of children age 6-11 years with obesity: 17.7% (2011-2012)
- △ Percentage of children age 2-5 years with obesity: 8.4% (2011-2012)

Since the coddled, "fluffy," and emotionally in-touch approach to reality very obviously doesn't work, we deliberately took the opposite approach. Our approach is about "facing up reality" and about who's responsible for the size, shape, and overall health of your body. It's entirely about **YOU** facing-up to taking responsibility for **YOU**! We're focussed entirely on solutions which work, and

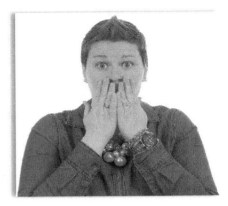

about getting you into the best shape possible, and as quickly as possible.

If someone is offended by our approach, and in facing up to "them" actually being responsible for the size and shape of their own body, then they and everyone who agrees with them are part of the problem. The problem I refer to is one which has created a society where many people believe it to be impolite to simply "tell it like it is," and state the obvious. More importantly, being offended at facing the fact that everyone is directly responsible for the size and shape of their own body, has created a society with a serious obesity epidemic.

### Responsibility, Willpower, and Body Shape

When we talk about responsibility, willpower, and body shape, we should clarify that we're talking about people who weren't born disabled. Nor are we talking about those who have suffered physical injury and are disabled as a result. We're also not talking about people who have a **GENUINE**, and we stress the word **GENUINE** medical condition which they had no part in deliberately creating.

People who don't fall into these categories, or into similar, **GENUINE** categories which we haven't listed, then by default they fall into a category which many people might not enjoy facing up to. The category of people who must take responsibility for the size and shape of their own body and health.

It's an inescapable fact that if you don't fall within a category listed in the paragraph above, then **YOU** have deliberately chosen the current size and shape of your body. It's simply stating the obvious. We believe that many people want to deny the obvious when it comes to their body weight, simply because the reality of it all is much too painful. Tough! Reality is always going to be reality, despite what you might want to believe. If you're athletic and muscular, then you've almost always deliberately chosen to be athletic and muscular. If you've developed exceptional flexibility, then you've almost always chosen to deliberately develop exceptional flexibility. If you decorated your home so that it has pink walls, then you deliberately chose to have it painted pink. None of these decisions were made by accident, or by your pet dog, or cat. The list could go on...

Therefore, almost **EVERYONE** who is overweight or obese has almost always deliberately chosen to be overweight and obese. If this is you, then, the reason why you have deliberately chosen to be overweight or obese, or to have whatever body size and shape you currently have, is because of the following:

- ⚠ **YOU CHOOSE** the type of food and drink which you consume.
- ⚠ **YOU CHOOSE** how much food and drink you consume.
- ⚠ **YOU CHOOSE** how often you eat and drink every day.

▲ **YOU CHOOSE** if you eat either highly processed foods or natural unprocessed foods.
▲ **YOU CHOOSE** if you exercise or not.
▲ **YOU** can **CHOOSE** to learn how to exercise if you don't already know how.
▲ **YOU CHOOSE** to read the labels on food products, or not.
▲ **YOU** can **CHOOSE** to learn how to understand the labels on food if you don't already know.

You may notice a theme developing here. The theme words are: "**YOU**," and "**CHOOSE**." If you're overweight, you can't blame anyone else for that. No one forces you to consume more food and drink than you need to maintain a steady, healthy, and lean body weight. You make the deliberate choice to place the food in your mouth. You make the deliberate choice to chew the food. You make the deliberate choice to swallow the food. No one forces you to do this. Equally, you also make the choice of either performing a basic exercise routine on a regular basis or not. Only you can make that choice.

In respect of willpower, we accept that to make certain choices might require you to have and to exercise a strong willpower. However, this is the same for everyone. **YOU** are not an exception to this basic fact. Willpower is the differentiator to success and failure in everything in life. Everyone who uses the "willpower" excuse, in that it's always harder for them, and it's somehow easier for others to exercise willpower, is just making another pathetic and obvious excuse for their own weakness and failure.

Willpower is the crucial factor in how Olympic and other record-holding champions are made. Their success doesn't just "happen" to them by accident. These people battle with their willpower every moment of every day, and in ways, most people can't even begin to imagine. This is especially true when they train through physical, mental, and spiritual pain barriers to achieving sporting greatness.

At an even higher level, members of the Elite Special Forces such as the Special Air Service regiment (S.A.S.) take willpower and determination even further. For anyone who was raised in the proverbial "vacuum bottle," and who doesn't already know about the S.A.S., here's a brief outline.

The S.A.S. was formed in 1941 before the United States had even entered World War 2. The S.A.S. are the original Special Forces regiment, from which all other special forces have been modelled. For example, Delta Force was formed in 1977 as a direct result of Anglo-American military cooperation. U.S Colonel Charles Alvin Beckwith was seconded to the S.A.S. in the UK to learn their methods, with the intention of forming the 1st Special Forces Operational Detachment-Delta, AKA: Delta Force.

The S.A.S. have the toughest and most challenging testing selection process in the world. Many of those who try to pass the infamous "S.A.S. selection" fail to do so because they literally die in trying. If someone passes "selection" to join the S.A.S., then they've already demonstrated having exceptional physical abilities, together with extraordinary mental aptitude. More importantly, they've also demonstrated having almost beyond-exceptional determination and willpower.

This is only the beginning, at this stage the S.A.S. soldiers begin to face even tougher tests in real combat situations. Challenges which might include being dropped miles behind enemy lines, typically in a 4-man group, running 35+ kilometres overnight while carrying a 120lb+ pack, engaging an enemy who usually greatly outnumber them in a firefight, perhaps rescuing hostages, before eventually being extracted to safety. The list of challenges which S.A.S. soldiers face on a regular basis could go on and on, and they have already filled a plethora of books with them. However, among the many qualities someone needs to possess to become an S.A.S. soldier, perhaps the most crucial are: willpower and determination.

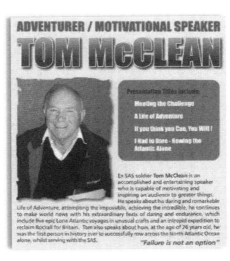

I'm proud and privileged to know a former S.A.S. soldier who exceeded even the exceptionally high standards set by the S.A.S.: Tom McClean. Tom's ethos is simple: "Failure is not an option." Tom made history in 1969, and captured a World Record in the process, in becoming the first man to row the Atlantic Ocean solo. In 1982 Tom took another World Record by sailing across the Atlantic Ocean in the smallest boat, measuring just 9 feet 9 inches in length. When his record was broken by someone sailing the

Atlantic Ocean in an even smaller boat, Tom demonstrated his ethos: "Failure is not an option" by chainsawing two feet

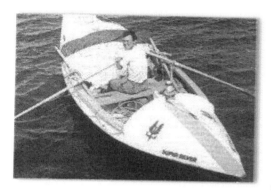 off his own boat to make it just 7 feet 9 inches in length, he then sailed the Atlantic Ocean in it and regained his World Record. Tom's list of extraordinary achievements could go on, and it is well worth visiting Tom's website to read more about his extraordinary achievements at: motivationspeaker.co.uk.

Does any of the above come easy to Tom McClean, and others like him who earn the right to join the S.A.S., or any other Elite Special Forces unit? Are these people just somehow "lucky?" Are they born "lucky?" Tom McClean certainly wasn't born "lucky," because he was abandoned as a baby and raised in a tough orphanage. Are these people just naturally blessed with a special willpower? No, of course not, and you're kidding yourself if you think they are. It's no easier for any of them to exercise their willpower and determination than it is for anyone else. In fact, it's considerably easier for you to demonstrate enough willpower to simply control the type and quantity of the food you eat, than it is to do anything even close to what Tom and other members of the S.A.S. have achieved.

The reality is that we're not even suggesting that you do anything which is exceptionally challenging and hard. You're not being asked to row the Atlantic Ocean solo in the smallest boat or pass S.A.S. selection. The most you need to do is exercise enough willpower and determination to make better food choices, eat less, and take a little exercise. This isn't rocket science. If you're someone who whines, moans, and complains about not having enough willpower to simply eat a little less, or to take regular exercise, try putting it in perspective in respect of what's a real challenge, and what's not. You're not a special case, and you're not unique in the fact that it's not always easy to make the right choices. Just like everyone else, you must take responsibility for the decisions you make. The sooner you face the reality of these facts, the sooner you'll begin to succeed in taking control of your body shape, your weight, your fitness level, your strength, and your life in general.

Your success in everything in life is all about the choices you make every day. The same choices we all face about exercising our willpower and determination when we need to. The choice to either succeed or fail in life. My Father always impressed upon me that if one human could achieve something, then so could I. This was because I was no different than anyone else. The only thing that would always differentiate between my success and failure, would be my deliberate choice to exercise willpower, determination, and good judgement.

## *Making Positive Choices*

In our opinion, the "career" excuse makers should be especially ashamed of themselves, and their pathetic "pity party" approach to life. If they aren't already inspired by extraordinary people like Tom McClean, then they could do well to learn about another shining example of inspirational courage and determination, the amazing Sam Rafowitz.

I first met Sam, and his wonderful son, several years ago when I performed a TV interview which was to be

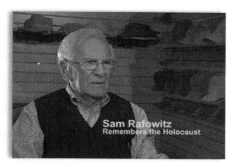

included in Steven Spielberg's Holocaust Memorial Archive. This picture here is from that interview.

Sam is a Holocaust survivor. He was a young man in his mid-teens when Hitler invaded Poland, triggering the start of World War 2. Unfortunately, the vile Nazi invaders soon rounded-up Sam, his Mother, and the rest of his family, together with many other completely innocent people. Why? Simply because they were Jewish.

Sam was first interned in a hard-labour camp, and then eventually in concentration camps. In fact, during World War 2, Sam had the very questionable "privilege" of being interned in every concentration camp that Hitler's Nazis ever built. After D-Day in 1944, the allied forces slowly but surely liberated Europe. In doing so, they would occasionally find one of these well-hidden camps, and liberate the prisoners held there. Unfortunately for Sam, every time the allies got close to liberating a concentration camp where he was interned, the Nazi commanders would simply transfer Sam, and all other able-bodied prisoners to another camp, much deeper inside the Nazi-occupied territory. They did this so that they could keep using them for slave labour as long as possible, in the ridiculous hope that in doing so they could also keep the Nazi war machine alive, and somehow win the war.

The last camp where Sam was interned was Bergen-Belsen. This was the same camp that Anne Frank was also interned in. The amazing diary of Anne Frank wrote about life under Nazi occupation became one of the most famous books of the 20th century. Bergen-Belsen didn't have gas chambers. However, between 1941 and 1945, the Nazis still managed to murder over 70,000 innocent people held prisoner there.

During the many years in the death camps, Sam and the other prisoners were violently abused every day. Unbelievably, vast numbers of innocent people were tortured to death in unimaginably sick ways, simply to amuse the vile Nazi commanders. All prisoners interned there were mercilessly starved of food, being fed on only the absolute minimum of rations. In fact, when Bergen-Belsen was eventually liberated, over 13,000 bodies were found of people who'd died from starvation alone. During my TV interview with Sam, he recalled that before Bergen-Belsen was finally liberated, he'd eaten nothing except grass for over 2 weeks.

The question is: with no apparent hope in sight, how could anyone possibly maintain a positive mental attitude while enduring these unimaginable horrors for years on end? Sam told me that he managed to remain positive because he deliberately CHOSE to remain positive.

At the time he told me this, his words surprised me a great deal. However, the more that I thought about it, the more that I realised that what Sam had said made complete sense. Sam realised that if he wasn't murdered, then the choices he made every moment of every day would ultimately determine if, and how, he would survive.

Over the years as a fitness and strength coach, I've exchanged some strong words with many excuse makers who chose to blame the size and shape of their body on sickness, depression, and going through "tough times." Tough times? Sickness? Depression? Seriously? When compared to the amazing Sam Rafowitz, and many of others like him, most people, and especially the "excuse maker" types have zero concept about what is genuinely tough, or not. The excuse makers have about as much comprehension of a tough time, sickness, or depression, as Adolf Hitler had about how to be a compassionate humanitarian. They have ZERO comprehension.

In deliberately choosing to remain positive, and as healthy as possible, under the most adverse circumstances imaginable, Sam's deliberate daily choices literally made the difference between life and death. More importantly, after he was liberated by the allies and nursed back to health, Sam didn't use the horrors that he'd been through as an excuse why he couldn't achieve things. After the war was over, Sam built a business empire from nothing except the skills he'd learned by making caps and gloves out of dead prisoners' clothes in the concentration camps. As a prisoner during the war, he did this initially to help himself, and to help others survive the bitterly cold winters they faced in Eastern Europe. After the war was over, and Sam eventually relocated and settled with his family in Minneapolis, Minnesota, USA., where he could use these same skills to help even more people. Through hard work and determination, Sam's initial tiny cottage industry of making caps and gloves grew to become a multi-million-dollar business.

It was also a business which provided much-needed employment for several thousand people over the years. Ironically, all the people which Sam employed had endured none of the hardships and torture that Sam had endured. These people all started out in life in the safe environment of the Mid-Western United States, and with much more money and opportunity than Sam ever had when he first started. The key difference between Sam and the people who worked for him, was simply a matter of willpower, determination, desire, taking responsibility for his own actions, and in making deliberate, positive choices every day.

Today, at the time of writing this book, Sam is in his late 80's. However, due to him consistently making good choices and exercising willpower and determination, he remains slim, sprightly, extremely active, healthy, and comparatively fit. When we look around at other people of a similar age to Sam, we almost always see frail, infirm, and elderly people. This makes me wonder just how many of those people preferred making excuses about why they can't exercise, and if made deliberately bad food choices, instead of exercising willpower and good judgement. When it comes to making excuses for why you can't do something, the person who always ultimately loses is the person making the pathetic excuses.

## The Starvation Diet Excuse

In telling the story about the amazing Sam Rafowitz, it's clear that everyone who was interned in a concentration camp was subjected to a near-starvation diet. Obviously, starvation diets are unhealthy, and we'd never recommend them for any reason. We also realise that for most people it's not considered to be politically correct to even mention this subject. Therefore, it's a good thing we've already cleared up the fact that we're not especially politically correct.

Without a doubt, making people suffer near starvation during World War 2 was completely sub-human, and vile. It does highlight one of the most pathetic excuses made by exceptionally stupid people. This is when they try to convince others that they eat "almost nothing," and yet they remain fat and overweight.

Fact: During World War 2 many people were forced to suffer near-starvation diets. In doing so, they were eventually reduced to an emaciated physical condition, it's just a physical inevitability. When people say things like: "I eat hardly anything, and yet I simply can't lose any weight," then they literally insult the precious memory of the millions of innocent people who starved, and suffered, at the hands of the Nazis and others like them.

What do the stupid people who say this really think happens? Do they think that "the food fairy" comes around each night and makes them absorb fat through their skin? Or do they think that they gain weight, and stay fat, by simply looking at too many pictures of yummy food? Hello? To coin a well-known phrase from a sci-fi show:

"You canna' change the laws of physics." Similarly, you can't change the laws of biology either. You don't get fat, and stay fat if you genuinely eat "nothing." If you've ever said anything even remotely like: "I eat hardly anything, and yet I simply can't lose any weight," then every time you utter those stupid words, all you achieve is to make yourself appear to be completely stupid.

I've always actively supported the survivors of the Holocaust in many ways, including financially. I was even made an honorary member of the Jewish community in my hometown of Manchester, England in the late 1970's.

## HELEN WRITES

I openly admit to having said these exact words throughout the years as another one of my famous "plexcuses."

I can't even count the times I've uttered the words: "I eat hardly anything, and yet I simply can't lose weight."

I had no idea how many calories I was consuming. A handful of M & M's here and there or a small piece of chocolate 2 or 3 times throughout the day.

I did eat three times a day, but those three meals were probably in the 800-1200 calorie range per meal and then include the little snacks of chocolates I am sure I was around 4000 calories or more.

## Chapter3: *You Are What You Eat*

Good nutrition accounts for approximately 80% of your success in body shaping, athletics, and bodybuilding. If you get that part right, then the physical training aspect is comparatively easy.

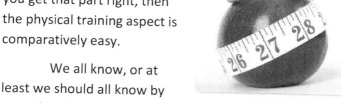

We all know, or at least we should all know by now, that it's not good to eat junk food, sugar, high fructose corn syrup, meats, dairy products, foods high on the glycaemic index, and simple carbohydrates. Similarly, we should all know by now, that high fibre foods are generally good for us. They help to maintain a clean digestive tract, eliminate toxins and fats, as well as help you to feel fuller and more satiated after eating.

While most people seem to broadly know these things, the most common disconnect most people seem to have is about what their body is composed of, and where it gets the construction material it needs from. Some people completely fail to make the connection that the physical material their body is composed of, and replenished with, is directly made up from the food and drink they consume. I've no idea why this "disconnect" exists, even amongst supposedly intelligent people. Perhaps it's connected in some way with the mechanism that prevents certain people from accepting that they are responsibility for themselves, and the health, size, and shape of their body.

I often wonder what these people think happens to the food they eat? Where do they think the source material comes from which their body uses to create their muscle, fat, skin, bone and hair? Do they think that their body somehow miraculously grows on its own and that the food they eat has absolutely nothing to do with it? Perhaps they do, in some peculiar way.

Even after these people understand the basic fact that their body's composition is directly made up from the food they consume, they still seem to have trouble with another obvious fact. This is that, if they eat low quality, highly processed junk foods, then that's all that their body's "construction engine" is given to work with. The

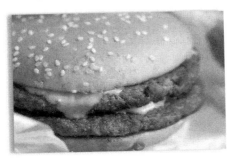

composition and overall appearance of their body will reflect that fact.

It's just common sense that if you consume junk food, then your body composition will consequently be composed of whatever it can extract from that junk food. Since some people have a hard time processing this very simple concept, I'll use a few analogies to help.

Firstly, let's take the analogy of you having to construct a new house. If you deliberately bought only low quality, basic grade materials to construct your new house from, how surprised would you be if your new home developed constant, and sometimes serious structural faults? Next, if we shift the analogy to that of a car, and how your business depended upon you building a brand-new car to sell, but you deliberately chose to only buy the lowest grade metals, glass, and electronics. How surprised would you be if your new car was constantly plagued with parts failures and warranty issues, which eventually caused you to lose your business? Alternatively, if you had to construct an aircraft, and then fly in it over the Atlantic Ocean, risking certain death if your aircraft failed, would you deliberately construct it from only the lowest grade materials possible? Lastly, if you were the manager of a racehorse capable of winning millions in cash, would you deliberately feed it on only low-grade junk food, and never have it exercised properly?

Surely, you'd never do any of these things, or allow any of them to happen if your money, your life, or business depended upon it. Not even someone who demonstrates the intelligence level of an average pet Labrador dog would do it. Amazingly, people do this sort of thing to themselves daily and think nothing of it. Just look at the size of the junk food industry. This offers a clue as to how people across the western world have been brainwashed into not associating the fact that they are the physical result of what they eat.

Similarly, if you consume the infected flesh of animals, then your body will process the infected flesh and it will construct and repair your body with whatever it can extract from it. In some cases, with animal infections such as B.S.E. or Bovine Spongiform Encephalopathy, human consumption of infected meat often resulted in a painful death. Let's not forget the fact that it was originally thought that B.S.E. couldn't be transmitted from beef cattle to humans. It is my belief that the scientists who originally took this position, were probably encouraged to do so by the farming industry to try and protect it from the full financial impact of the crisis.

These things aren't rocket science to understand. How does anyone know exactly how many of the animals that are used to make up the human food chain were sick or infected when they were slaughtered? They don't know, that's the unpalatable answer. There are millions of animals slaughtered every day to feed people, and you can bet for certain that there is quite a high percentage that didn't die in the best of health. People simply don't want to think about these things, and that statistically, a lot of the animal flesh they've eaten during their lifetime has almost certainly come from animals that have been suffering from cancers, infections, and many other nasty diseases. Scientists simply don't know what the long-term effects are of repeatedly consuming infected animal flesh. It seems that only time, and resultant new human diseases, will tell. These are horrible and inconvenient truths to face. However, facts are facts, despite what you might want to believe. It's part of the overall axiom that: "you are what you eat."

These are just some the reasons why vegetarians, and especially vegans, are generally much healthier than people who eat meat. Statistically, they suffer from far fewer ailments, and they tend to live longer than non-vegans, and especially the heavy meat eaters. If you're not already a vegan, then it's highly likely that on the day that you read this section of the book, then you've already consumed the flesh of an animal that was sick or ill when it died. Furthermore, if anyone is concerned about how to

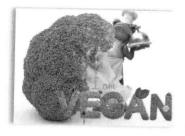

get enough protein if they don't eat meat, then they don't need to worry, because they'll get more than enough in a vegetarian or vegan diet. Even though it has never been widely publicised, some of the most massive, strongest, and most successful bodybuilders have also been vegetarian or vegan.

The silence about these things is probably because supplement manufacturers and magazines want to sell as much cheap dairy-based protein, and desiccated liver products as possible. They make massive profits from consumers who buy into the myth that the best kind of protein supplements are animal based. They especially love the dairy-based derivative protein supplement, whey, because it's cheap and they can make massive profits from selling it wrapped up in marketing hype. There will be more information about this, and vegan protein sources in the later section about dairy.

## *Pill-Popping*

My first-hand experience of life in the USA has revealed a society that believes it's perfectly normal to take medications daily. Somehow, people have become convinced that

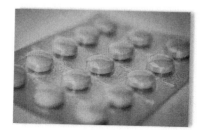

what's needed are palliatives, instead of resolving the root cause of the physical problem they're suffering from, which is usually diet related.

It's highly amusing to watch the TV commercials for medications that contain numerous warnings about all manner of side-effects, some of which are very serious and include the possibility of death.

We're both shocked at the numerous TV commercials we've seen that lead the viewer to believe that heartburn, and acid reflux, are somehow "normal," and people need to always be prepared by having some of their medications to hand.

No one seems the slightest bit interested in resolving the cause of the problem. Instead, they're almost entirely focussed on masking the physical manifestation of the condition.

In respect of something as simple as heartburn or acid reflux, what about simply modifying your diet, and excluding the foods that are known to cause heartburn and acid reflux? That would completely resolve the problem without the need for any medication, and there would be no nasty side-effects either.

If you eat something which causes acid reflux and heartburn, then it's simply common sense that whatever you're eating isn't good for you. You are what you eat, there's no escaping that fact. It's really that simple.

I would like to share my experience with medical issues. In my early 40's I was diagnosed with acid reflux, and the doctor then prescribed a medication to help the symptoms.

Thinking back to that time, what is shocking to me is that the doctor never once told me I should change my diet. He just prescribed a pill! I took the pill daily and it did help, but as soon as I missed a day I would get the acid reflux again. I certainly did not want to be on medication the rest of my life. Once I finally lost the 40 lbs I also realized that I did not need to take the medication anymore, my acid reflux was gone. I can clearly see now that you are, only and always composed of what you eat.

I also remember a time when I was frustrated with my weight, and I went to see the doctor for some advice about how to lose weight. His response was quite shocking. Unbelievably, he told me not to worry about it. He also told me that women typically gain 10 lbs each decade, so I should just expect to keep gaining, and that for my age I was just fine.

I am 4 feet 11 inches tall, and at 147 lbs, that made me clinically obese. I was very discouraged when I left the doctor, and it motivated me to prove him wrong! I didn't want to accept the fact that I would be that overweight and uncomfortable for the rest of my life.

### Are Humans Really Omnivores?

When the subject of a plant-based diet arises, almost immediately, the first thing that people bring up with glee is that if you examine the teeth of a human adult we're omnivores, simply because we all have the remains of what were once much more pronounced 4 canine teeth.

In short, this is laughable. People who simply use the remains of what were once 4 canine teeth as their sole argument as to why we're anthropologically designed to be big meat eaters are just demonstrating how a little knowledge can be both dangerous, and completely misleading.

The eminent anthropologist, Dr Alan Walker, of John Hopkins University, Maryland, U.S.A. led one of the first modern research teams to extensively examine this often-contentious subject. The results of the study were startling and were published in detail on May 15, 1979, in the New York Times.

Since then several other extensive studies on the same subject have been completed, with the results of all of them drawing the same conclusions. Evidence to support this has even been found in the stomach contents of early humans who have been found frozen in the ice until recently.

Through the process of studying the fossilised remains of teeth, bones and joint structure of Australopithecus, our early human ancestor, it became clear that they were not, as was once thought, predominantly meat eaters.

Early humans didn't even eat a great deal of grass, leaves, shoots, and they certainly weren't omnivores. In the 12 million years that it took Australopithecus man to become Homo erectus, the primary diet was fruit. This is because early humans, and modern humans, are not omnivores, we're frugivores.

More importantly, human biology and physiology haven't changed in this brief period of "anthropological time" and we simply gradually have adopted omnivorous eating practices. However, just because we've adopted these practices, it doesn't mean that they're good for our health, because they're not.

Modern society has made it become customary for humans to consume meat with almost every meal. This has reached the point whereby that for most people, eating meat is now a habit and one which is hard to break. It's even hard for many people to comprehend that we're simply not naturally "designed" to eat meat and that eating meat is making them become gradually increasingly ill from all manner of ailments.

The way in which most people react when it's merely suggested that humans aren't designed to eat meat is nothing short of being ridiculous. However, if a pet dog could tolerate being forced to eat fruit and vegetables in equal proportion to that of meat with every meal, the same people who can't seem to comprehend that humans aren't designed to eat meat would completely baulk at the idea feeding a dog in that way. They'd believe it was simply wrong to force-feed a dog, or any other animal, a diet which is unnatural for it, even if the animal in question could tolerate the diet well enough not to become immediately ill from short-term consumption of fruit and vegetables. Why is it so different for humans?

To demonstrate why we humans aren't designed to eat meat, and why we're frugivores, not omnivores, I'll examine the entire human digestive tract from beginning to end. This will include the teeth and jaw structure, and even the process of getting our food into our mouth to begin the journey through our body.

Compared to omnivores and carnivores, humans have soft hands and pathetically weak nails. Our fingernails couldn't possibly be used as a tool to catch, tear, and cut flesh. Instead, they're the simply the remnants of a moment in pre-history, nothing more.

The human jaw structure is that of a frugivore, which is nothing like that of an omnivore or carnivore. The jaw of an omnivore or carnivore has no lateral movement which is needed to chew and grind plants, whereas the human jaw moves forwards and backwards, side to side, as well as up and down.

The teeth of a true omnivore comprise of long, sharp and curved fangs, with short and pointed incisors, and molars which are a combination of both flattened and blade shaped to aid in cutting meat. Human teeth are completely different, and we already know how pathetic our so-called canine teeth are. Human teeth are the same as all other frugivores, with incisors that are short, flattened and shaped live a shovel, and with molars that are flattened, and feature modular cusps. For most people today, the remains of these once briefly canine teeth are almost indistinguishable from those surrounding them.

Human stomach acidity is in the region of pH4 to 5 when food is in the stomach, the same as other frugivores, whereas the stomach acidity level of an omnivore with food in it is either less than, or equal to pH1.

The process of peristalsis in a human is the same as that of other frugivores. Peristalsis is the involuntary symmetrical constriction and relaxation of the muscles of the intestine. They propagate in a wave-like motion down the intestinal tract, and it forms an integral part of the waste elimination process. In omnivores, this process doesn't require fibre to stimulate the process, whereas, in humans and other frugivores, fibre is essential to stimulate the process.

This is something that I always find amusing when observing the dietary habits of western nations, and especially people in the United States. Somehow, the processed food industry there seems to have brainwashed much of the population with clever commercial advertising into believing that taking fibre supplements is the "normal" thing to do. Why do so few people stop to think for a moment that this is complete nonsense? To anyone who exercises any kind of independent thought, it's blatantly obvious that taking a fibre supplement of pill simply isn't "normal" and certainly isn't needed if the food people ate was plant-based, nutrient-rich, and naturally fibre-rich as it should be.

The human circadian rhythm, AKA sleep pattern, is to sleep for approximately 8 hours or less during each 24-

hour cycle, the same as other frugivores. Omnivores and canines both follow a pattern of between 18 and 20 hours of sleep during each 24-hour cycle.

Humans must extensively chew their food, just like other frugivores. Omnivores and carnivores either swallow their food whole, or they perform only simply crushing before swallowing.

Human brain chemistry is fuelled by glycogen, just like other frugivores. The brain chemistry of omnivores and carnivores is fuelled by proteins and fats.

Humans can only process Phytosterols which occur in plants, just as other frugivores and humans can't naturally process cholesterol from animal sources. Omnivores and carnivores can, both metabolize and process, large amounts of cholesterol easily and efficiently.

Human colon length is long, with the small intestine being approximately 9 times longer than the length of the body, and the digestive process typically takes between 12 and 18 hours. This is the same as other frugivores. Omnivores and carnivores have a short colon, which is only between 1.5 and 3 times the body length of the animal. The digestive process of a carnivore takes between 2 and 4 hours and an omnivore between 6 and 10 hours. This means that when a human consumes meat, it remains inside the body long enough to begin to rot and putrefy as it passes through our long and complex intestinal tract. Since this is the case, and since meat and dairy products contain the sugar Neu5Gc which is alien to humans, and which always causes some degree of immune-response inflammation, then it shouldn't be surprising why this begins the entire process of making us ill.

The list of how humans compare almost exactly to frugivores, and not to omnivores, could be much longer, and fill several more pages. However, I'm sure that by now you either get my point, or you never will, either way, it's excellent "food" for thought.

## General Advice for Weight Loss

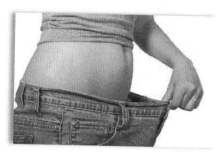 The best way to achieve a proportionate physical appearance is always going to be by not allowing yourself to become overweight in the first place. That may sound almost too simple, but it's a fact.

The real differentiating factor between those who gain weight to the point of becoming obese, and those who don't, is about personal standards of what weight, and body shape is acceptable, maintaining an objective perspective, self-image, and how they feel. No one who is obese became obese overnight. That doesn't happen. It's up to the individual concerned to decide when it's time to stop gaining weight and reduce the amount of food they eat. It always takes time to gain weight, so it's not hard to spot when it's happening. When you gain a little weight, your clothes become tighter, until they reach a point when they don't fit anymore. At that point, it's like a fork in the road, and a life-changing decision must be made. Do you buy new, larger size clothes, or do you cut back on your food intake and lose weight?

If you make the decision of buying new clothes, when you're existing clothes feel too tight because you've gained too much weight, then the process will probably repeat itself. it becomes likely that you'll be repeatedly buying larger size clothes, to replace the ever-tightening ones in your wardrobe. In addition, you need to stop blaming the tumble dryer for shrinking your clothes and own up to the fact that you're gaining too much weight.

## HELEN WRITES

*This was one of my favourite "plexuses." I own up to the fact that over the years I used this "plexcuse" literally 100's of times, maybe even 1000's! My advice is to be honest with yourself, especially if you have used this "plexcuse" yourself.*

Basically, weight loss is an easy concept to understand, and it's an easy thing to achieve. If weight loss is your goal, then you first need to determine exactly how many calories you need to consume each day to maintain a steady body weight. You do this by simply adjusting the quantities of food and drink you're consuming until you find the right balance. Keeping a detailed food diary really helps this process, and don't expect to find the balance too quickly. It's probably going to involve a little trial and error.

To begin with, document as much detail as possible about everything you consume each day for a period of between one and two weeks. List everything in fine detail, and then research how many calories are contained in

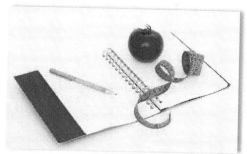

what you've consumed. In addition, list other details about the nutritional values of your food and drink. One of the best ways we've found to track your daily food intake is by using an excellent application called www.myfitnesspal.com. It's free, and it's easy to use. However, most people are completely shocked when they begin tracking and documenting everything they consume over a period of two weeks. It's almost always far more than what they originally thought.

## HELEN WRITES

*When I first started tracking my food intake, I was stunned to find that it was consuming more than 4000 calories a day! At a height of only 4 feet 11 inches, it's no wonder why I felt so completely unfit, lethargic, and was clinically obese.*

Once you have all the information about what you are consuming, then you can adjust the quantities, type of food, and the calorific values of what you consume until you find the balance-point to maintain a steady body weight. When you've eventually determined your personal balance-point, then you can simply adjust what you eat to either make you lose or gain weight. It's really that simple.

Even though the basics of weight loss, and weight gain, are just common sense, all the companies that sell diet plans, and weight loss supplements, want to make you believe that it's a much more complex and mysterious subject than it is.

In life, and especially when it comes to diet and exercise, we don't believe that anyone is truly lazy. Instead, we prefer to believe that they simply lack proper motivation. None the less, many people just don't seem to want to make the effort and begin logging their food intake, let alone experimenting with eating more, or less food, until they find their weight-loss/gain balance point.

For the best advice on making wise food choices, weight control, and eating to improve your overall health, we recommend exploring the 'Forks Over Knives' nutrition books, cookery books, and their excellent website. These resources contain all the information needed about nutrition to help create a new, and healthier "you." In addition, the website and books contain lots of great recipes to prepare delicious, healthy, and nutrient-rich meals. Go to: http://www.forksoverknives.com/

We also recommend that you should also explore the research papers, publications, and the general advice of the following outstanding nutrition experts:

⚠ Dr Caldwell Esselstyn
  (http://www.dresselstyn.com/site/)
⚠ Dr T. Colin Campbell (http://nutritionstudies.org/)
⚠ Dr Alona Pulde & Dr Matthew Lederman
  (http://www.lifestylemedicine.org/LMMB0909)
⚠ Rip Esselstyn (http://engine2diet.com/)

In our opinion, the people listed above, together with the rest of the "Forks Over Knives" team, are the best possible source for good advice on healthy eating, weight loss, weight control, eating for athletic success.

## You Can't Flex Fat

The next thing we want you to impress upon you, and encourage you to remember forever, is that: **YOU**

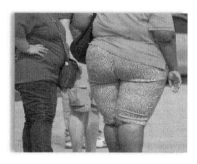 **CAN'T FLEX FAT.** This should be obvious, even to those who seem to have an I.Q. beginning with a decimal point. However, many people just don't seem to understand this basic rule, unless it's driven home with a proverbial sledgehammer. Since you can't flex fat, this means that the only way you can shape your body is to tone-up your muscle structure. In doing so, both men and women must build a little muscle in the process.

That last statement will probably come as a huge shock to many women. Only the non-existent "gods of exercise" know why this should typically be the case, but sadly it is. We don't know how many times we have heard women say, "But I don't want big muscles, I just want to tone." Sorry ladies, this is just another pathetic excuse not to exercise. It's just a fact that most women do not have nearly enough testosterone in their bodies to build "manly" muscles. What building a little muscle tone will do, is enhance your feminine shape.

The following question may sound completely ridiculous to everyone who is not a lifetime member of, "The Society of Village Idiots". It's a ridiculous question that I've been asked once too often. The question is: *"How long will it take to exercise to turn my excess fat into muscle?"* Seriously. People have asked this utterly ridiculous question much more often than one might think. Just in case you don't already know the answer, I'll clarify matters: YOU CAN'T TURN FAT INTO MUSCLE. They're two completely different substances, and if you didn't already know this,

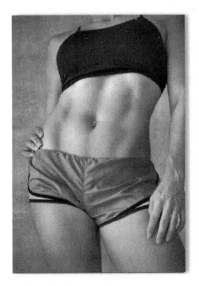

then you may need to take another look at what you studied at school.

The only way we can think of possibly turning fat into muscle is by becoming a wizard through attending the fictional "Hogwarts School of Witchcraft and Wizardry," just like the great J.K. Rowling's character Harry Potter.

What you need to think about doing with your excess body fat, is burning more of it. This way you'll eventually reduce it to a point so that you'll begin to reveal much more of what's underneath, which is muscle.

Before I go any further talking about body fat, and how it should be kept under control etc., I'd like to first take a closer look at what fat is, what it does, why we need it, what it's used for, and what happens to fat on its journey of expulsion from the human body.

Fat is a substance that is often written about in books and articles on diet and exercise. It's often seen as the "enemy" we all face in one way or another, however, is it really? No, of course, it's not. Fat is an important part of our overall body composition, and without it, we'd die.

As we know there are several types of basic fat in humans, and some the differences between the main types we're dealing with.

A. There is fat under the skin which is called, subcutaneous fat. This fat which is between the skin and the muscle prevents the muscular 'definition' from being visible which you can often see in athletes.

B. There is fat cosseting and surrounding our internal organs, which is called visceral fat. This fat which rests in the cavities between organs contributes to excess belly size and to the general appearance of being overweight.

C.  There is fat interspersed with muscle which is called, intermuscular fat.  This fat within the muscle itself has the visual appearance of marbling, such as in the streaks of fat in the cuts of meat you can see in supermarkets.

D.  There is epicardial fat which is a form of visceral fat which is deposited around the heart which might significantly affect cardiac function in various ways.

E.  There is bone marrow fat which inside our bones.

F.  There is ectopic fat which is the storage of (supposedly) small amounts of triglycerides in tissues such as the liver, heart, pancreas, and skeletal muscle.

G.  Finally, there is brown fat which is a special type of fat that is primarily stored around the neck and the large blood vessels of the thorax to effectively act in heat exchange and body temperature regulation in cold weather.

Obviously, there is much more to fat than one might at first think.  In relation to diet and exercise, we're primarily concerned about not allowing our body to carry too much fat so that we lose our muscular shape, and head towards being obese.  We also primarily think about fat as a reserve of lipids which can be oxidised as a form of energy to meet the physical demands we place upon of our body during physical activity.  However, this is only a small part of the overall process.

Some people mistakenly belie that since we burn only a comparatively small amount of our fat reserve as energy, the rest must be somehow excreted from the body through our intestinal system and colon.  In fact, the only food that is ingested that passes out through your colon is undigested dietary fibre. Everything else you ingest is simply absorbed into your bloodstream, then into your organs and, after that, it passed out of the body as CO2 (carbon dioxide) and water.

That's right, as you breathe you exhale the CO2, and the water part mixes into your circulation to eventually be excreted as sweat or urine. The only way you can increase the amount of CO2 that you exhale is by moving your muscles during some form physical activity. There are also other processes that come into play such as increasing your BMR, or Base Metabolic Rate, through exercise and lifestyle changes. However, when a triglyceride (fat) is burned up (oxidized) the process consumes a large number of oxygen molecules and produces CO2 (carbon dioxide) and water (H2O) as the waste products of the process.

Therefore, to lose weight one should move your body more through general activity and exercise, eat less than your body needs to remain overweight, and generally exhale more.

## *Food Labels*

The best thing that people could do to help them make better food choices when shopping is: **ALWAYS READ AND LEARN TO UNDERSTAND FOOD LABELS.** We can't stress this one simple point strongly enough. This is because it can make getting into shape, staying in shape, and eating healthier, a much easier process. Many foods undergo processing techniques and have contents added to them which makes them nothing short of being complete rubbish. Food which few people would even feed to their pets.

We've noticed that TV commercial advertising techniques for pet foods in the United States has taken the approach of having pet owners compare the contents of pet food labels side by side, to see which they'd prefer to feed to their pets. Invariably, when these people read the food labels, they always choose the brand which contains the most natural, and unprocessed food materials. We'd love to see a human food manufacturer take the same approach in their advertising. However, we don't think that this will happen in our lifetime, because most of them simply wouldn't be able to sell their products ever again once people knew and understood what they contained.

Perhaps the more important question is: "Why don't people read and compare the food labels for the foods they feed themselves, and their families in the same way?" We've no idea why this is. Since people don't usually read food labels, and if they do, then most don't even understand the basics of what they mean, it also means that they're usually feeding their family some very nasty stuff. We could fill a whole book about this subject alone, so we'll keep it brief to help us make our point in this respect.

Many food manufacturers produce foods which they want to appear to be "healthy," however, they're anything but healthy. This is because they have added lots of things like hidden sugars, fats, dairy, and even chemical food additives. The most obvious things to look for on a food label are things like calories, fat content, salt content, and proteins etc. You want to avoid high-calorie, high-fat foods, with little or no protein content.

You should take note of the order in which the ingredients are listed on a food label. This is because the order, or content/quantity of material, is in descending order, from high to low. The items that are first on the list, are always in greater quantity than the items last on the list.

You want to avoid all foods which have been processed or heavily processed. All chemicals in food will have a side-effect of some sort, it's just a fact, and almost none of them are there for the good of your overall health. They're there to make it easier for the manufactures to make foods be more taste-addictive and have a longer shelf-life. The faster a food will turn bad in storage, then the more natural it is, and the better it will be for you.

Many foods such as peanut butter will contain something called hydrogenated oil, and other hydrogenated or partially hydrogenated items. These are all incredibly bad for you. Hydrogenated oils are natural oils such as palm oil, or soybean oil, and which are then turned into something quite remarkable through the processing they receive. To create a hydrogenated oil or a partially hydrogenated product, the first thing they do is to heat it, to between five hundred and one thousand degrees, while under several atmospheres of pressure. They then add a catalyst such as nickel or aluminium, to the oil, and continue to "cook" it for several hours until a chemical reaction takes place. The molecular structure of the oil eventually changes, and instead of it being liquid at normal room temperatures, it becomes either partially liquid or a total solid. This is now either partially hydrogenated or fully hydrogenated oil.

Once it has become either partially hydrogenated or fully hydrogenated oil, it is only ONE molecule different to a plastic. These products have been proven to be harmful to your health, and yet it somehow remains a legal food additive. Unbelievable!

For example, peanut butter often contains either partially hydrogenated or fully hydrogenated oil, which makes no sense when it can easily be made without the use of these products. Costco's own brand of peanut butter is excellent. It contains only natural ingredients and ZERO hydrogenation. If Costco can produce a really great product like that, then why can't other brands? The answer is that they can. We believe that the reason they choose not to is that they put their profits before the health and welfare of their customers.

Sugar is another hidden additive in many processed foods. When you check the ingredients list on the label for anything ending in "ose," it should be a warning. This includes names like glucose, maltose, sucrose, fructose, and lactose. These are all forms of sugar, and with the latter being also a dairy product.

It's also worth looking for other forms of sugar such as honey, treacle/molasses, rice syrup, agave, and of course the dreaded high fructose corn syrup. They're all bad for you, and they're extremely high in calories.

High fructose corn syrup, or HFCS, is one of the worst, and one of the most common ingredients found in western foods. High-fructose corn syrup is a mixture of simple sugars called monosaccharides. High-fructose corn syrup contains more fructose than any of the other sugars, so it's basically much sweeter. Therefore, it has a massive effect on your insulin levels, and it creates a chain reaction. Research has confirmed that high-fructose corn syrup can directly cause you to overeat, and therefore gain excess weight more easily.

This is because your body contains a hormone called Leptin, and our body uses this hormone to decide if we have had enough to eat. It's known as "the satisfaction hormone," and we'll cover these two hormones in more detail in the next section. High-fructose corn syrup travels directly to your liver, and therefore, avoiding the Leptin which would trigger a reduction in your appetite. If you consume too much high-fructose corn syrup, it causes your Leptin signalling process to malfunction, and the result is that you eat more of the foods containing high-fructose corn syrup as you attempt to satiate your appetite. The result of this is increased body fat. Since the farming industry has such a powerful political lobby, the producers of high-fructose corn syrup have somehow managed to get laws changed to hide it more cleverly on food labels. We'd recommend doing regular online searches for the latest name it is being allowed to "hide" under. These names include to benign-sounding terms such as: "natural sweetener."

Lactic acid is a surprisingly common dairy-based food additive. It can be used either as a preservative, or as an acidity regulator, and it's found in a wide variety of foods. If you're avoiding dairy products, then check for this in foods such as baked goods, confectionary, ready meals, salad dressings, and savoury products.

"It's an 'E' number so it must be bad for me, right?" Many E numbered food additives aren't especially good for you, however, there are also some which are. One such number is E322. This is a code name for lecithin, which is a natural substance present in all living cells, including nerve and brain tissue. Soybean lecithin is a common food supplement taken by fitness enthusiasts, and bodybuilders, because it protects the cell membranes, and the polyunsaturated fats within the cells, from oxygen attack. It's also a good synergist to antioxidants in fats and oils.

## The Hunger Hormones – Leptin and Ghrelin

There are two hormones which our body produces which are commonly called "The hunger hormones." These are Leptin and Ghrelin.

Leptin is a hormone produced by fat cells, and its role is to decrease your appetite to ensure that you don't overeat and store too much body fat as a result.

Conversely, Ghrelin is a hormone which increases your appetite, and it encourages you to eat when your body decides that you need more nourishment or more stored body fat for emergencies.

Both hormones form part of your body's appetite regulation system, and they work as part of a larger and more complex regulatory system, which includes your stomach's density receptor mechanism.

When you're slim and have a low percentage of body fat, your levels of appetite-suppressing Leptin are naturally less. This is because you have less of the body that is needed to physically produce the Leptin hormone.

However, there are some people who develop a resistance to the appetite-suppressing effects of Leptin.

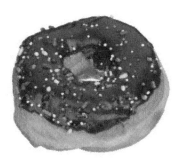

More importantly, some research now indicates that Leptin helps to regulate Ghrelin production, your appetite increasing hormone. The latest research suggests that your body can become "accustomed" to being fat. This means that because you initially allowed yourself to become fat, and then stay fat for long enough, this may have created a state where your body is so fat that it is preventing you from losing weight.

If the Leptin hormone signals the brain that your body has stored enough fat, this begs the question: "if Leptin is produced by your body fat, then why don't fat people get slim, because if they have more fat, then they should automatically produce more Leptin?" This is a good question, and the answer is surprising. Research shows that if you've allowed yourself to become fat to the point of obesity, and to remain obese for long enough, then you could eventually develop a form of Leptin-resistance.

In clinical studies, animals were fed in such a way that it caused them to become overweight. They were then given artificially high doses of additional Leptin. To begin with, the animal's appetite became markedly, naturally suppressed. The result was that the animals initially began to lose fat. However, this effect only lasted about two weeks. After that time, they seemed to develop a form of Leptin-resistance, which then caused their appetite to increase, and for them to gain weight again.

There could be a similar effect taking place in humans. The people who have initially allowed themselves to become overweight to the point of obesity maybe remaining overweight and obese because they had allowed themselves to become overweight in the first place. People may have trained their body to become Leptin-resistant. Therefore, being "fat" has become their new "normal." The subject of Leptin-resistance is obviously a highly complex issue, one which needs much more research. However, the following factors all play a role:

- Not exercising.
- Over-exercising.
- Overeating.
- Insulin level cycling.
- Lack of quality sleep.
- Stress.
- High fructose corn syrup AKA: HFCS/ fructose syrup.
- Snacking.

The Ghrelin hormone causes your appetite to increase. It's primarily released in your stomach, and it sends the signal to your brain that you're hungry. Naturally, your Ghrelin levels are highest before you eat.

Unsurprisingly, these levels gradually reduce while you're eating, and then continue to reduce immediately after you've eaten.

This is a good reason why you should eat your food slowly, and why you should allow your food to digest a little before eating more. The process of producing Ghrelin to signal your brain that you're starting to get full is always delayed, when compared to the immediate feeling of being hungry. Therefore, if you don't eat slowly, and allow your food to digest a little, you could easily end up overeating. We're sure that almost everyone will remember their Mother telling them as children to: "eat slowly and to chew their food properly." Well, surprise, surprise, your mother was right.

Naturally, if someone is under-eating, then research has also shown that Ghrelin levels will naturally rise. Likewise, when someone is obese, Ghrelin levels will usually fall. Research also indicates that Ghrelin's part in your appetite control 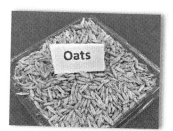 mechanism may be much more complex than it was originally thought. This research has indicated that a diet that is higher in complex carbohydrates and protein, help to suppress Ghrelin production much more effectively than diets which are higher in sugars, saturated fat, processed foods, high fructose corn syrup, and simple carbohydrates. Eating highly processed junk foods will leave you feeling hungrier than you would be, if you'd eaten more unprocessed, natural foods.

Sleep also helps to regulate your body weight and fat content. People who are sleep deprived are typically those who will produce higher levels of Ghrelin.

Research clearly shows that exercise, and your BMR, or Base Metabolic Rate, plays a big part in decreasing any Leptin-resistance you may have developed. It also plays a part in suppressing your Ghrelin production.

It all comes back to the simple and inescapable fact that your deliberate choices, directly determine the size, shape, and overall health of your body. Your deliberate choices also have a direct effect on health-related problems, because of you being unfit, overweight and obese. Everyone must take responsibility for what they eat, and for how much they eat. If you've already allowed yourself to become fat and obese, all is not lost. You simply must demonstrate higher than average levels of determination to break the bad habits you've developed, and to make the positive changes you need to make. Getting into shape will be tougher than if you hadn't helped to create your own problems, to begin with. However, with willpower and determination, you can and will succeed. When you do eventually succeed, you'll win the respect of everyone around you, especially fitness professionals. They will understand just how much extra willpower, courage, and determination it's taken you. Therefore, we strongly encourage you to start now, and we wish you success beyond your wildest imagination.

## Lipoprotein Lipase and Insulin

The main reason why most people regain any weight they lose after following a diet plan and training regimen is due to deliberately poor lifestyle, and food choices. There may be other factors which also need to be considered. Recent studies have shown that after a period of weight loss there is a certain protein in our bodies that is created in higher quantities. Furthermore, it also can help undo all the weight loss you've achieved to date.

It's a hormone called Lipoprotein Lipase, and its job is to move fat, AKA: triglycerides, into your fat cells. This entire process becomes much more efficient when your levels of insulin are higher, therefore, it's part of the reason why insulin stimulates the storage of body fat.

The latest research studies have shown that doing as little as only 3 minutes of super-high intensity exercise

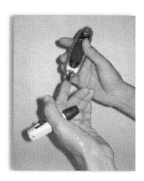 per week can improve insulin sensitivity between 24% and 35%. After a workout, your body will be more sensitive to insulin. This means that it's easier for your body to transfer the sugar in your bloodstream so that it can be stored in your muscles where it can be used as fuel. Insulin also affects how efficiently your body synthesises protein, and physical exercise is one of the most powerful methods you have available to help you normalise your insulin level.

Insulin sensitivity is important to keep the blood sugar stable because when you eat and begin to digest your food, glucose is released into your bloodstream. This triggers the release of insulin to absorb the glucose. The greater your sensitivity to insulin, means that your body will

require smaller amounts of insulin to lower blood glucose level s. This is when compared to someone who has low insulin sensitivity, who will require more insulin.

Extremely low insulin sensitivity is known as insulin resistance. This is a condition which results in high levels of insulin, glucose, and damaging fats circulating in the bloodstream. It's important to note that you can also be too sensitive to insulin, which can cause some other equally damaging problems. These include damage to blood vessels, diabetes, obesity, osteoporosis, high blood pressure, heart disease, heart failure, cancer, and can be a driver for general weight gain. Periods of both stress and illness introduce short-term periods of reduced insulin sensitivity. In most cases, insulin sensitivity should recover once the stress or illness has passed.

Insulin isn't the only factor that helps Lipoprotein Lipase become more efficient, the physical action of losing weight does too. Your body is anthropologically designed to store higher levels of fat than we 20th-century humans find desirable. Over thousands of years, humans developed a sort of self-preservation fail-safe mode. This means that when your body senses there might be a food shortage, it triggers mechanisms and processes that help your body to store more of whatever food it can, to preserve your life. Naturally, your body stores the food as fat, which is needed for energy.

Carbohydrates, and, simple carbohydrates that make up most of what's contained in junk and processed foods, all have an enhanced effect when it comes to increasing your insulin levels.

Fruit juices aren't great when it comes to weight control, because they release sugar (fructose) into the

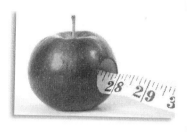

bloodstream much faster than if you ate a piece of fruit. This is because a piece of fruit contains natural fibre, which buffers the rate which the sugar is released. The result of drinking fruit juice is that it dramatically increases your insulin level to combat the ingestion of so much sugar.

This can be a problem when it comes to growing muscle, and bodybuilding. This is because it is often forgotten that to achieve this, you need to consume more carbohydrate than protein. The reason is simple, muscle is composed of only 22% protein at best, with the rest being water, carbohydrates and fat.

What do you do if your muscles need carbohydrates, and yet at the same time, carbohydrates also increase your insulin levels, which in turn can increase your ability to put on more body fat? The answer is simple, it's a combination of making deliberately good food choices and portion control. Complex carbohydrates digest

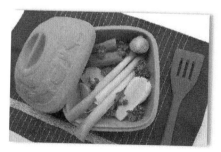

much slower than the simple carbohydrates, and sugars, contained in junk food. This means that they release sugar into the bloodstream at a much slower rate than the junk food does.  Complex carbohydrates don't increase the levels of insulin in your blood as fast, or as much, as the simple carbohydrates and sugar in junk foods do.  Therefore, complex carbohydrates should make up the majority, or your carbohydrate food choices, and you should try to avoid all forms of junk food.

Portion control is an essential element of all diets and eating plans, especially if you want to maintain a leaner, more muscular body for the long term.  It's better to eat several small meals each day, rather than eat one or two large ones.

## HELEN WRITES

*I suffered from this for many years.  I would want to lose weight, so I would skip breakfast, but by lunchtime, I was so hungry I would eat everything in sight!*

*Then I'd wait until dinner time, and once again I would be so hungry that I would be snacking on whatever I could get my hands on, until supper time when I would usually have 2 and 3 helpings.*

*Along with all the wrong food I was eating, I was also eating only 2 or 3 times a day, with huge portions at each meal, totalling a whopping 4000+ calories a day.*

*I would always eat fast, so when I did eat, it went down so quickly that by the 3ʳᵈ helping I would feel like a beached whale!  Then I would tell myself tomorrow will be* better, but of course, it wouldn't, and the cycle would begin all over again.

From the start of training under the direction of my coach, he put me on a strict meal plan consisting of 6 meals a day, and I was advised never to skip a meal. He also stressed how important it was to plan ahead.

Once I'd got myself prepared with a list of the best food choices, and a workable eating plan, I was ready and set to go!

Food preparation was the biggest issue I had to contend with, and it certainly wasn't my strong point. In fact, the first time I prepared my meals in advance it took me almost the entire day.

I reserved each Sunday as preparation day, and even though it initially seemed like to be a chore, as the weeks passed, it all got easier.

I also realized the importance of eating 6 small meals a day. That way you never let yourself get too hungry, and because of this, I could go the entire day without ever over-indulging during any one meal.

It was also helpful for me to track all the food I ate on the MyFitnessPal app. That app works exceptionally well, and it also really makes you think twice before you grab a piece of chocolate or a full sugar soda drink.

Once my competition was over, the hardest part was realizing that I had a wider variety of food choices when compared to the 8 weeks before my competition.

*I now use the macro system for my food choices and portion control. Using the macro system of deliberate food choices and portion control, it's now given me a much greater degree of freedom and enjoyment in maintaining a level of body fat, and a much easier way to do it.*

*Furthermore, the macro system of deliberate food choices and portion control also means that I'm usually only between 4 and 6 weeks away from being in peak contest condition, and the period leading up to the contest is much more pleasurable than before.*

## *The Glycaemic Index*

By following a low Glycaemic Index diet as part of your overall eating plan is an excellent way to maintain levels of body weight, and especially body fat, which is especially important to anyone involved in sports, serious athletics, body shaping, and bodybuilding.

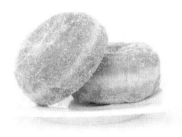

The Glycaemic Index (GI), is a number associated with food. Food types fall into 3 categories of Low Glycaemic Index with a score of 55 or less, Medium Glycaemic Index with a score of between 56 and 69, and High Glycaemic Index with a score of 70 and above.

The Glycaemic Index score indicates the food's effect on a person's blood glucose, AKA: the blood sugar level. A score of 100 represents the standard marker which is the maximum possible and is the equivalent of pure glucose. Therefore, the Glycaemic Index is useful for calculating how much of the available carbohydrate is in any given food choice you make.

Complex carbohydrates with a low Glycaemic Index marker of 55 or less, are digested, absorbed, and used by the body at a slower rate than those foods with a higher Glycaemic Index marker. They don't cause a rapid rise in insulin levels, or for overall levels to rise too high. Food may contain other components that also contribute to the overall rise in blood sugar and aren't measured as part of the Glycaemic Index.

The Glycaemic Index marker represents the total rise in blood sugar following the consumption of each type of food. However, it doesn't necessarily consider how quickly the level rises. The steepness of the rise can be influenced by several factors, such as the quantity of fat eaten with the food. Choosing to eat only certain complex carbohydrates and other healthy foods with a low Glycaemic Index marker help in the management of weight loss, and overall weight management, as well as in controlling diabetes. They also reduce the risk of developing type 2 diabetes and other diseases. Foods with a low Glycaemic Index marker of 55 or less:

- Fruit - not fruit juice.
- Beans
- Most grains
- Most nuts
- Mushrooms
- Seeds
- Oats
- Barley

⚠ Rye
⚠ Most vegetables

Foods with a medium Glycaemic Index marker of 56 to 69:

⚠ White sugar
⚠ Fruit juice
⚠ Enriched wheat
⚠ Bread
⚠ Pita bread
⚠ Pumpernickel bread
⚠ Unpeeled boiled potatoes
⚠ Raisins, prunes
⚠ Bananas
⚠ Ice cream

Foods with a high Glycaemic Index marker of 70 and above:

⚠ Glucose
⚠ High fructose corn syrup
⚠ Sweet potatoes
⚠ White bread
⚠ Bagels
⚠ Most white rice
⚠ Most processed breakfast cereals

## *Success Doesn't Always Taste Sweet*

Now we all know that consuming excess sugar will

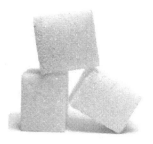

increase your insulin level, and lead to weight gain.  You should also know by now that consuming sugar in your diet will dramatically increase your chances of developing both diabetes and heart disease.   New discoveries have revealed that sugar can even attack your core DNA. It was quite shocking to read the results of a 2008 scientific study about this. In the study, scientists exposed the brains of test mice to high levels of sugar for only 6 hours. Not an especially long period of time. However, the results of the experiment were dramatic. The excess sugar exposure for only that short period of time, still caused epigenetic changes to the DNA of the mice, with long-term damage being the result.

This means that the choices that you make every day in the foods you eat can have an epigenetic effect on your body. Your food choices can directly turn on, or off, your fat gene, your diabetes gene, or even your cancer gene. Dairy foods and the milk protein casein have been scientifically proven to be directly responsible for turning on, and off, cancer production. This isn't great news for dairy-lovers, and especially for those who take whey protein supplements. We'll explain more about this in a section entitled: "Inconvenient Truths About Dairy."

## Protein 101

In a fitness, body shaping, and bodybuilding lifestyle, one of the first things most people think about is protein. There's probably no surprise there. Especially since we've all been taught at school that protein is essential to our growth and that it's especially important in the growth of lean muscle.

Even though protein is an essential dietary element, there are limits to both the amount we need and to how much we can absorb at each meal. There are also limitations because of the strain on the liver in the processing of the by-products which are produced from consuming protein. Therefore, it's a generally accepted wisdom that it's best to eat some protein with each meal, rather than consume your daily intake all at once.

To better understand the overall concept of protein, and how much we really need, I'll use an analogy. Imagine a highway which is designed to accommodate a certain number of vehicles to function freely, and flow smoothly. Increase the number of vehicles in this analogy, because just like in exercise and protein consumption, more is always better, right? What happens then? Does the highway continue to function freely, and flow smoothly? No, of course, it doesn't. Just like your body in relation to exercise, protein, and many other things in life, it can only handle a certain quantity of anything before it becomes congested, sluggish, and gridlocked.

Current research indicates that the optimum amount of protein the average human should consume with each meal should be an absolute maximum of around 30 grams. It also indicates that an average person who doesn't exercise should consume about 46 grams of protein per day for women and 56 grams per day for men.

However, once someone gets into the fitness, body shaping, and especially the bodybuilding lifestyle, the quest for increasing their protein intake becomes almost an obsession for most people. The Academy of Nutrition and Dietetics reports that bodybuilders require about 0.63 to 0.77 grams of protein per pound of body weight each day and that 1.4 to 1.8 grams of protein per kilogram are required to build muscle mass.

However, this obsession for increased protein consumption is typically fuelled by misguided, and poorly trained coaches. In addition to this, the obsession is also fuelled by the myriad of confusing magazine articles and advertisements, which all promote the supposed need to consume massive amounts of protein.

Many people read the glossy magazine articles about nutrition and supplement requirements, and then take them to be "science-fact," as if they were reading a reputable scientific journal. They simply fail to understand that the terms, words, and phrases that are used in relation to protein, and other supplements in these 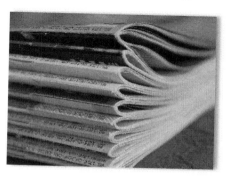 articles, are usually very cleverly worded to make their allusion to science data **appear** to be science-facts. The only real facts in these articles are that they **allude** to certain conclusions. Furthermore, the articles usually contain no reputable, non-biased, independent scientific data as you'd expect to find in a proper university study about the subject.

People also fail to realise that these articles are usually very clever forms of **paid** advertising by the supplement manufacturers, published under the guise of being independent editorial content. With dramatically falling magazine print sales, publishers had to find a way to compensate for their losses. They did so by allowing an increasing number of "supplement manufacturer friendly" journalists, or even the manufacturers themselves, produce heavily biased editorial content for their magazines. Look for yourself, and you'll see that these articles are almost always surrounded by a great many glossy advertisements for the supplements written about in the editorial.

With this sort of "infomercial-journalism" taking place in the hard-core bodybuilding and fitness magazines, it's not surprising that people are easily drawn into believing the myth that they need to consume massive amounts of protein to achieve the success they desire. When I hear the so-called "experts," and "coaches,' who extol the virtues of taking massive amounts of protein, one of the first things I automatically ask myself is: "What products are they selling?" Almost invariably every one of them is selling some sort of nutrition supplement, or they're a multi-level marketing agent/representative for a nutrition supplement system that isn't sold in stores.

Unfortunately, when it comes to building muscle, there are some inconvenient truths that must be faced when it comes to protein. Aside from the fact that human muscle is not made up entirely of protein, there's another highly inconvenient truth which isn't talked about by protein supplement manufacturers. This is that consuming excessive amounts of protein causes kidney damage. When too much protein is consumed, the kidneys must deal with it before expelling it from the body as waste via urine. Over time, people who consume too much protein and especially animal-based protein, risk the permanent loss of their kidney function.

Since there's been a great deal of deliberate confusion generated about what we call "the protein myth," mostly by supplement manufacturers, I'll wind the clock back to where it all began. This way we can take a more objective look at what protein is, what it does, and then how much you really need.

Protein is an essential part of all living organisms, including body tissues such as muscle, and hair, etc.

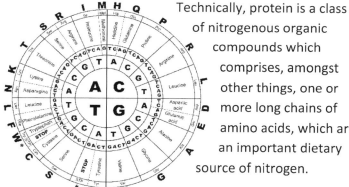

Technically, protein is a class of nitrogenous organic compounds which comprises, amongst other things, one or more long chains of amino acids, which are an important dietary source of nitrogen.

**Amino Acid Wheel Chart**

Most plants and other organisms are able to biosynthesize all 20 standard amino acids. However, humans and other animals are not. This is because the enzymes that synthesize certain amino acids simply aren't present in humans, or other animals. Therefore, humans and animals must obtain the 9 amino acids they can't synthesise from what they eat from other sources. The amino acids that humans and animals can't synthesize are known as "essential amino acids."

In 1839, a Dutch chemist from Utrecht, Gerardus Johannes Mulder, described the chemical composition of what we now call protein. He claimed that albuminous substances are made up of this common substance. He was the first person to isolate it and used the name, protein.

This was a word first used by Jöns Jacob Berzelius in 1838, and comes from the Greek word "proteios," which means "of primary importance." The first protein was isolated from meat, which directly led to 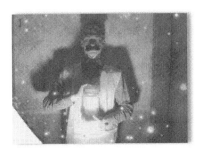 the idea that meat and protein were basically the same things, and that "meat makes meat." However, in a publication by Jöns Jacob Berzelius (1779-1848) he pointed out that animals draw most of their protein from plants. Unfortunately, this important point was somehow overlooked from that time onwards, and for most people that mistaken belief still survives today.

In the late 1800s a German chemist, physiologist, and nutritional scientist, Carl von Voit, found that the amount of nitrogen in excreted urea (urine) is a direct measure for protein a human body is processing. Since he taught at the University of Munich, he had a significant influence on other budding nutritionists of the day. It is von Voit, who is now considered by many to be the "father" of modern dietetics. He was also the first to recommend that the average adult male should consume over 100 grams of protein per day.

In retrospect, it's interesting to note that when this was eventually published, von Voit had already made additional discoveries leading to new recommendations about how much daily protein is needed. His new research showed that the average male only needed about 52-55 grams of protein per day to be healthy, and later research showed that even lower levels should be recommended. Amazingly, the highly inaccurate initial recommendations continued to be promoted, and the myth was born that the average adult male should consume between 100 and 140 grams of protein per day.

Since many of the people who promoted von Voit's initial ideas were also von Voit's students, and with some of those having already become prominent in their field, it only served to cement and perpetuate the original misconception. From that point onwards, when any contradictory evidence was presented which suggested that less than the original estimates of protein was needed, it was automatically dismissed without any further thought.

Later, a breakthrough study at Yale University by Professor Russell Henry Chittenden, who some believe is the "father of American biochemistry," clearly showed that male students performed consistently better in their physical training if they consumed what was accepted as being a low protein, mostly plant-based diet.

In 1909, Osborne and Mendel's work with amino acids eventually led to the discovery that there are 9 essential amino acids which humans need to consume. Around the same time, the Connecticut Agricultural Experiment Station completed a detailed review of vegetable and seed proteins. This was done under the leadership of Thomas Burr Osborne, who was a biochemist. Incidentally, he was also the co-discoverer of Vitamin A. Subsequent research revealed that the 9 essential amino acids aren't exclusive to animal-based proteins, they're originally found in plants and they're then found in the animal-based products, such as meat because the animals ate the plants.

Despite the research clearly showing that plants also contained protein, it was summarily dismissed by closed-minded so-called scientists, probably through their prejudice and scientific arrogance. In doing so, many people then made yet another astounding mistake in their assumptive conclusions, by calling plant-based protein "low quality." More importantly, they did so without any scientific data to support their arrogant and stupid dismissal of the conclusive findings.

The only data they had and cared about to draw their conclusions from was that gram for gram, plant-based protein didn't promote as much bodyweight gain as animal-based protein did. They didn't even stop to consider what kind of weight was gained. People just automatically assumed that weight gain from animal sources protein is automatically a gain in lean muscle mass, which isn't true.

Scientific arrogance, ignorance, and prejudice continued. Even though some of the initial research data measured amino acid sources and protein efficiency ratios, etc., it was still flawed and biased. Furthermore, it didn't even report the fact that research clearly showed that there was a direct effect, in respect of increased cancer growth, from the consumption of animal-based proteins and dairy products.

Eventually, other researchers examined the composition of human muscle tissue. It revealed something which was quite remarkable. This was that human muscle is composed of between 16% and 25% protein, depending upon the research study type of the sample used. However, most research averaged between 20% and 22%, with the rest of the muscle being composed of around 70% water, carbohydrates, and fat. Therefore, eventually, the more enlightened scientists, researchers, and eventually even bodybuilders, began using the actual physical composition of the human body itself, not voodoo-based myths, as the real guide to what nutrition an athlete requires.

One of the strongest, and most massive bodybuilders of all time, Mr Olympia Mike Mentzer, took this data and then based his own successful diet on the facts, not the myths. He believed in a diet comprising the bulk of the calories he ingested of between 50 and 60%, carbohydrates, rather than from excessive quantities of protein. Plenty of water was also important too.

The logic behind this reasoning was simple. The research showed that the average human, under optimal training conditions, and without the use of drugs, can only usually gain about 10lbs of muscle per year. Since one pound of muscle contains 600 calories, 10 lbs of muscle mass equate to a value of only 6000 calories.

Therefore, logic and science clearly show that only an additional 6000 calories need to be consumed, spread-out evenly daily throughout the year, to gain all the lean muscle that it's possible for a human to gain.

That averages to only 16.44 extra calories per day. More importantly, only four of those calories needs to be from a protein source, which is because muscle is approximately only 20-22% protein by composition. Surprise, surprise! Mother Nature's foods already had the natural nutritional balance right after all.

In addition to this, the famous, and eminent sports scientist, Dr Ellington Darden, gathered research data that supported this concept. Since that time, he has pointed out on many occasions that it's water and carbohydrates that are the most important components of building muscle, not protein. Again, this is simply because of applying logic about water and carbohydrates being the bulk of what human muscle is composed of. Dr Ellington Darden's advice to some of the greatest and most successful bodybuilders of all time was to consume a diet of between 60-70% carbohydrates, 15-25% fats, and 15-25% protein. Therefore, he advised that a 200lb bodybuilder should consume about 0.36 grams of protein per 1lb of body weight, in other words about 72 grams.

He is also directly quoted as saying that: "Magazines only "big-up" protein for marketing purposes and financial gains. This is because they cannot make money pushing complex carbohydrates as calories. and plain water, to their readers." This is probably a universal truth, that many people who read those magazines completely forget about.

With clear scientific evidence like this, it's amazing why many so-called coaches and bodybuilders, are still so obsessed about consuming massive quantities of protein. It makes absolutely no sense.

If the tissue you're seeking to build isn't composed of anything more than about 22% protein, then it's stupid to literally stuff yourself with massive quantities of protein, in the pathetic and misguided belief that "more is better." The logic and the science all point to feeding your body according to the proportion of elements which it's composed of, and not by force-feeding it unnaturally excessive quantities of any one element.

More importantly, consuming too much protein will slow down your body shaping and bodybuilding progress. This is because your body will be desperately trying to process the continued protein overdose it's being force-fed.

Here it is in the most basic terms, with simple analogies that even the most prejudiced, and stupid "gym-rat" can understand. If you were mixing condensed food that required adding water to make the meal complete,

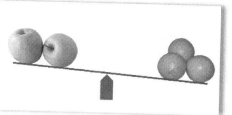

would you add more water than recipe-ratio required? No of course not. If you did, then you wouldn't get the desired results, and you'd ruin the recipe.

In another analogy, if you're asked to mix cement which has a critical cement to water ratio, would you arbitrarily double the amount of cement, just to be sure you got enough?  No, of course, you wouldn't.  If you did, then you'd mess up the whole mix and make it worthless.

So why do average "gym-rats," think the human body is any different?  We believe that it's because these people are easily "sold," and they haven't properly researched and/or understood the subject.

In fact, when we both first began training in gyms, even though it was decades apart and on different continents, we both noticed that most bodybuilders weren't just easily "sold," they were also very easily brainwashed.  We may be somewhat cynical in this observation, but we believe that most bodybuilders would literally eat horse poop if it was packaged correctly and someone who was a famous bodybuilding star endorsed it.

Now that we've established a few levelling facts about protein, and exactly how much we should consume as opposed to how much we're "sold" that we need to consume, we can explore another very significant point which we briefly touched upon earlier.

People haven't just been brainwashed about how much protein they need, they've also been brainwashed about the supposed benefits of animal-based protein over plant-based protein.  This concept is fully supported, perpetuated, and extolled by companies who want to sell massive quantities of cheap protein, such as dairy-based products.  After all, why not maximise profits - right?

The fact is, that research clearly shows that animal-based proteins, and casein, which is the protein found in all dairy products including whey protein, dramatically supports cancer growth.  It also supports general cardiovascular disease too. These effects are further enhanced in diets which are low in complex carbohydrates, and high in processed foods.

The question which most people ask at this point is usually something like: "How does eating meat and dairy products cause cancer?" This is a very good question. The fine details of the research findings of "the how and why" of the process are still emerging almost daily. However, it's a team of scientists from the University of California (San Diego) who seem to be leading the way with the current research on this fascinating subject.

For many years now, statistical and observational research has clearly shown an unquestionable direct link between cancer, and the consumption of dairy products and meat. Scientists eventually discovered more about how these foods directly influence the pH balance of blood after they've been consumed, and how acidic blood causes cellular inflammation.

The latest clinical research has taken this a step further. It indicates that the main reason why consuming dairy products and meat causes cancer is about a combination of a sugar molecule called N-Glycolylneuraminic acid AKA: Neu5Gc for short, how the human body perceives it, and chronic cellular inflammation which results from consuming it.

For dairy and meat-lovers, this sugar is found in almost all dairy and animal meat products. Despite what is commonly believed, human beings can only tolerate eating very small quantities of dairy products and meat, and once the tolerance threshold has been passed, which is currently believed to be only about 5% of a person's overall diet, then cellular inflammation takes place.

Humans can't naturally produce the sugar, Neu5Gc. Therefore, when it's absorbed into human tissue, the body responds to it as if it were an invader. It then activates an automatic immune response mechanism to combat it.

Scientists believe that this process, and the high levels of inflammation created by ingesting dairy products and meat, have a direct role in the development of the resulting cancers. The studies about this, and which have directly mimicked the actions of the human body when eating dairy products and meat, have proven conclusively to develop cancer in test animals.

The science is also clear in that animal and dairy-based protein causes serious damage to your body's endothelial cells. These are of vital importance to good health because they help to keep the arteries flowing freely. More importantly, **plant-based protein does not have the same adverse effect**.

In recent years, protein supplement manufacturers have exhorted the supposed value of whey protein to the point at which it seems to have gained almost mythical status. More worryingly, the supposedly fitness-conscious public happily bought into this myth and began spending huge sums of money on what is essentially a low-grade waste product.

It's a high-price rip-off, which the supplement manufacturers want you to believe is something very special, to help justify the grossly inflated retail prices they set for it. Through the mechanism of clever marketing, great advertising, and paid-for editorial infomercials, the supplement manufacturers have now created a massive industry from it.

If you've been a whey protein advocate, and bought into the myth, then you simply didn't thoroughly research the subject. As a result, you've been ripped-off into spending fortunes on a cancer-causing product that costs pennies to produce.

In addition to these significant problems, there's another factor to be considered: allergies. Dairy protein is one of the most common causes of stomach bloating and other allergic effects, with about 12% of the US population being officially lactose intolerant.

Lactose is a milk sugar comprised of two other forms of sugar, glucose and galactose. Most adults either completely lack, or they produce insufficient quantities of the lactase enzyme, which enables them to break down the lactose in dairy foods.

Therefore, without this enzyme, or with not enough of it, lactose is forced to be broken down by the bacteria in the lower intestines. During this process, the body's natural waste products combine with the lactose sugars, and they ferment. The result of all this fermentation is stomach distention, bloating, cramps, and even diarrhoea. Therefore, if you suffer from bloating after taking a dairy-based protein supplement, now you know the reason why.

You now know the facts. Get over what you've been "sold," and research the subject properly for yourself. Do it through reputable scientific journals, scientific publications, and studies carried out by research institutes and universities.

Don't do what many so-called coaches do and perform your research about diet and exercise by reading fitness magazine articles. No matter how scientific these articles appear to be, you simply can't rely on them. They could easily be clever infomercial-editorials supplied by supplement manufacturers.

We've now established that you really don't need to consume nearly as much protein as you've probably been doing. Even if you're an extreme strength athlete, you still don't need to consume huge quantities of protein, and if you do, then you'll simply slow down your progress because your body is trying to deal with the excess that you're misguidedly feeding it.

If you ate nothing else except a variety of fresh fruit and potatoes, then you'd still not become protein or amino acid deficient. To think otherwise is a myth because it's almost impossible to become deficient unless you completely starve yourself.

We'd strongly recommend that your protein requirements be supplied from plant-based sources such as legumes, which include beans (soybeans, black, navy, pinto, kidney, chickpeas etc.) peas, and lentils.

*I know what you are thinking as you read this, "Give up meat?! Are you crazy, no-way?!" I thought the same thing too when I first found out. I could never give up my beloved CHEESEBURGERS! I reluctantly first gave up Pork, then after a couple of weeks, I gave up beef.*

*I tried it for a couple of months and before you know it I no longer craved the beef. Then I finally gave up chicken/poultry. Each week got easier and easier. I would suggest giving up one meat group at a time. It made it much easier for me.*

*My dad would be turning over in his grave right now if he knew I gave up meat. After all, I was born into a family of hunters. Sadly, it is with deep regret that I also sincerely believe my father might still be with us today, had he only changed his eating habits, especially in respect of meat and dairy.*

In addition to the items already suggested, also look at consuming more nuts and seeds. There's a huge variety to choose from. They're all a great source of protein, and they're packed with many other essential nutrients.

Despite our research, we've still not been able to find a study which shows that even by consuming only the recommended minimum RDA of 10% protein, which is 10% of your overall daily calorie intake, it has any adverse effects on an athlete's muscle growth or sports performance.

Therefore, consuming plant-based protein within the so-called recommended mid-range, which is between 10% and 25% protein of your overall daily calorie intake, it is still more than enough to build muscle, even for a high-performance athlete. However, our personal recommendation would be to consume a maximum of about 22% protein, entirely from plant-based sources, and with a complete amino acid complex.

Scientifically proven data is hard to argue with. However, it's strange how some people simply "want to believe" something. even if it's not true. It's a phenomenon, just like in the famous sci-fi TV show where the FBI agent investigating paranormal mysteries has a poster on the wall which reads: "I want to believe." For some people though, no matter how much hard data is presented, they still prefer to believe the fairy tale. For some strange reason, these people seem convinced that if enough people believe something, then it must be true. They take comfort in the status quo. These are the same type of people also believe that the world is flat...

The problem with this fairy tale about protein is that if you choose to believe it, then it's not just your money that you're wasting, it's also your health that you're risking. You're risking the early onset of a variety of diseases, including cancer, impaired liver function, osteoporosis, heart disease, and a lowered metabolic rate. In addition, if you consume high quantities of animal-based protein, then you shouldn't be surprised that if one day, it has permanently adversely affected your arteries and it's found stored in your fat cells by doctors who are trying to save your life.

115

**Helen's Embarrassing Experience with Protein**

When I first decided that I wanted to get in shape and enter a bodybuilding competition, I knew I would have to change my diet. I was also "sure" that I would have to increase my protein intake, and start using whey protein, because that's what everyone who joins a gym or reads a bodybuilding magazine is told repeatedly.

I have no idea what I was eating in terms of my protein before I started a regular workout routine, but once I started hitting the gym six times a week, I increased my protein intake to about 20-30 grams of protein per meal, six times a day. Two of these meals consisted of 8oz of whey protein, and when added together with the regular food it totalled-up to feeding myself around 150 grams of protein per day. Over time, with a reduced calorie intake, and by following a good exercise routine, I successfully lost 40 lbs of excess fat which had plagued me for years.

In addition to this, I felt very accomplished by taking 2nd, 3rd and 4th place in my first Bikini Fitness Bodybuilding competitions. During those 8 months of hitting the gym six days a week, and in following the strict "accepted" meal plans, I had also suffered some side effects that I thought must just be "normal" for bodybuilders. One of the questionable side effects was that anyone I spoke with face-to-face could also tell what I had eaten that day. This was because my breath constantly smelled like a combination of

116

*chicken, broccoli, asparagus, or whatever other vegetables
I'd eaten that day.*

*What I didn't realize at the time was that was one
of the many side effects of eating too much protein. What
was worse was that initially, I'd no idea that I was suffering
from this problem, and when I eventually found out, it was
totally embarrassing.*

*I felt like I was in the best shape of my life, but no
matter what I did, breath-mints, or minty gum, you could
still smell my bad breath. I eventually resigned myself to
thinking that it was just something that I would have to
learn how to live with.*

*The other side effect I suffered was even more
embarrassing than the horribly bad breath. I suffered the
worst and the most continuous flatulence of my entire life.
Mercifully, I soon discovered that I wasn't alone in this,
because once you get to know them, bodybuilders will
openly tell you about the dreaded "protein farts."*

*Seriously? I looked super-hot by any standards, and
yet, in reality, I'd somehow turned into a bubbling gas
machine with added horrendously bad breath!*

*I remember one of the most embarrassing moments
was while I was walking through the gym near the end of a
workout. As I walked, I suddenly felt a dreaded "protein
fart" building in readiness to deploy!*

*I foolishly thought to myself that if I just let it out
silently as I walked, AKA: crop-dusting, then nobody would
notice. I couldn't have been more wrong.*

*After walking past a group of guys, turning heads as I did so, I eventually settled onto a nearby mat to perform my last exercise. That was when I heard those same guys who had just been flirting with me say to each other "WTF, I think the sewer just broke, go get the manager! It smells awful in here!"*

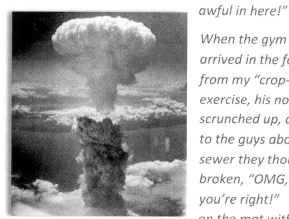

*When the gym manager arrived in the fallout zone from my "crop-dusting" exercise, his nose scrunched up, and he said to the guys about the sewer they thought had broken, "OMG, I think you're right!" I sat there on the mat with my face bright red and didn't say a word! There was no way I was going to own up and tell them it was me who had caused more devastation than your average biological strategic weapon.*

*My petite, yet muscular 4'11" and 105 lb frame might even be officially classified by the United Nations as a weapon of mass destruction due to my lethal protein farts, rather than being classed as a weapon of mass-distraction due to my stunning new body! Thankfully, no one ever found out that it was me who had caused the issue.*

*The other and more disturbing side effect I suffered from whey protein was stomach bloating. Overall, I was leaner than I'd ever been in my life, and yet after taking my "essential" whey protein supplements, I'd very soon suffer from some of the worst stomach bloating I'd ever experienced in my life. To make matters worse, the bloating was always the precursor to the onset of the dreaded protein farts. I was completely and utterly frustrated and bewildered. I looked the best that I had ever looked in my entire life, and yet at the same time, I didn't dare get close to anyone due to the damage I might inflict upon them!*

*After my competition, I met the veteran coach and internationally renowned fitness expert Brian Sterling-Vete. He immediately suggested that I do some research into protein, and the real science behind exactly how much someone should consume, even as a bodybuilder. What I found out shocked me completely. I was consuming around 150 grams of protein per day when the science clearly showed that a person of my size should only be consuming between 40 and 70 grams of protein per day!*

*From that point onward, I began consuming far less protein, and I immediately noticed that I no longer had bad breath! I could talk to someone without them knowing exactly what I ate that day! I also noticed within days of changing my diet that I no longer had the dreaded "protein farts!"*

*What a relief! Also, by switching to a vegan protein powder, I no longer had the bloating issues after drinking it. This was all just amazing in every way! Seriously, anyone who is trying to lose weight, get fit, begin bodybuilding or whatever it may be, the bad breath, the "protein farts" and the bloating are not normal! This is all part of your body sending you signals that something is not right.*

*I urge you to do your own research and see for yourself. I am so incredibly thankful that I did, and as I write I'm now training for my next competition.*

*Even though I'm consuming far less protein than before, I'm gaining much more muscle, I'm physically stronger, I look leaner all the time because I never get bloated, and I smell much better as well.*

*In addition to all of this, at the same time I changed my diet and dramatically reduced my protein intake, I also started training for my next competition using the ISOfitness™ system, which also means that I've dramatically reduced the length of time I spend training each day too!*

## *Protein Sparing*

One of the little-known bonuses of consuming carbohydrates is that they have a protein sparing effect. This means that they make even a comparatively low-level protein intake work with much greater efficiency. Your body will feel better, you'll be less lethargic, than if you continued to overload yourself with too much protein.

Protein sparing is the process where your body derives energy from sources other than protein, including stored body fat. Therefore, protein sparing helps to conserve your muscle tissue and reduce body fat.

The key to success in this respect is to maintain a healthy balance of complex carbohydrates in your diet, which are low on the glycaemic index, so that they help to provide the right balance of digestible energy, together with digestible protein.

Strength athletes and bodybuilders training will naturally create a state where their body requires, and preserves, the protein it needs to both repair itself and for new tissue growth.

However, contrary to what muscle magazines might want you to believe in their constant quest to sell you more protein supplements, consuming more protein doesn't enhance your protein-processing efficiency.

Therefore, if you want to get stronger and build bigger muscles, you need to eat more carbohydrates and consume only moderate quantities of protein.

## *Inconvenient Truths About Dairy*

The subject of dairy foods is a somewhat sensitive subject to most people. This is especially true when people are being told that their beloved dairy-based products are harmful to their health. For many years, cow's milk has been marketed to the public as being "healthy." It's been literally pushed onto unwitting consumers in the UK, Europe, and North America for decades. Today, it's become so ingrained in our culinary culture that it's seriously challenging to find foods, especially in restaurants, which don't contain at least some dairy products.

To get an objective overview of dairy, what it really is, and more importantly, how it affects the human body, we'll take a brief look at what cow's milk really is, what it contains, and what it does to the human body. In our opinion, the science-based facts you inevitably must face, make even the thought of consuming any kind of dairy product completely ludicrous.

121

*First, you must give up meat, and now dairy too?!? I know, it's crazy talk, but trust me, keep reading. For the record, these are all suggestions to lead a fitter, healthier life. You can take all, some, or none of the advice. It's up to you how you want to use the information we are giving you!*

Milk is a substance produced by a mammal to feed babies, and once they're old enough, they get weaned off it and move onto solid foods.

Most of the milk sold to the public in the west is cow's milk. However, in recent years several trendy sounding alternatives have entered the market. These include goat milk, sheep milk, lactose-free milk, and even buffalo milk.

One of the more shocking facts about cow's milk and one that is kept deliberately low-key by the dairy industry and the government is that all milk contains cow's blood.

When you drink milk or consume dairy products, you're drinking and/or eating the white blood plasma of a cow. Amazingly, the USDA allows milk to contain anywhere between 1 and 1.5 million white blood cells per millilitre of milk.  Furthermore, white blood cells in a place where they don't normally belong, are also called pus.

Therefore, in drinking cow's milk, you're actually drinking the pus of a cow.  Pus is something which forms at

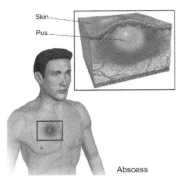

Skin

Pus

Abscess

Source: Blausen.com staff.
"Blausen gallery 2014."

the site of inflammation during bacterial infection. When it has accumulated sufficiently in tissue, it's also known as an abscess. Incredibly, researchers in California recently found 298 million pus cells in a single litre of cow's milk. When you stop for a moment and think about it, it's no wonder that the dairy industry is reluctant to make these facts widely known to the public.

In respect to breastfeeding, milk is excellent. However, this is provided you're a baby, and that it's from your own mother, who is obviously an animal of the same species.  Breast milk offers a great many benefits to the infant, in addition to the simple nutritional aspect of feeding.  These benefits include the antibodies which the parent has developed in their own body, and which are then transferred via the milk, to help the new baby fight-off viruses and bacteria.

What possible antibodies do humans of any age need, or want, from a cow?  Furthermore, since almost all cattle are given large doses of antibiotics, and some are also given additional hormones for various reasons, these will

123

also be passed on to the consumer of the milk, and via the associated milk by-products. Alarmingly, current laws do not force companies to tell consumers if they treat their cows with recombinant bovine growth hormone or rBGH. Furthermore, just because a dairy product has been labelled as being "organic." It doesn't necessarily mean that the animals that produced the dairy products have been grass fed. Besides, just because milk is organic, doesn't make it any less harmful to humans. Amazingly, the term "organic" typically refers to the processed "organic" feed which the animal has been given, and it tactfully ignores any antibiotics and hormones the animal has been given.

Since we know these things, an excellent question would be: "Do you really want to ingest the antibodies, antibiotics, and hormones, which come to you suspended in a milky liquid that is basically the white blood cells of a cow, or from any other species of animal for that matter?"

Osteoporosis is caused by several factors, with the most common being diet-related. Diets which are rich in animal-based proteins, and especially dairy products. This is because that when digested, these products increase the pH balance of your blood. In other words, they produce a state of highly acidic blood. Once the blood has become acid-rich, it must be neutralised before it causes damage to the infrastructure of the body.

Normally, consuming sufficient quantities of vegetables and fruit will neutralise most of the acid if the right balance of foods has been consumed quickly enough. However, this is almost always never the case. Western diets are typically woefully inadequate in this respect.

They can't be relied upon to neutralise the acidic blood caused by dairy and meat protein consumption. The body's next line of defence in neutralising acid-blood is for the body to find another acid-buffer. The most readily available acid-buffer for the body is calcium. Where does your body get the right source of readily available calcium? It can't get any from the undigested dairy products, therefore, your body naturally extracts it from your bones. Your body will basically dissolve your bones to produce enough alkaline to safely neutralise the high levels of acidic blood. More importantly, it continues to do so until your blood pH balance reaches a tolerable level again.

Dairy is a good source of calcium, right? Wrong! Dairy is a terrible source of calcium for humans. Where does a cow get the dietary calcium it needs? It gets it from the plants that it eats of course. Since many plants are an excellent source of magnesium, they allow the calcium contained in them to be easily digested, absorbed, and readily used by the body.

The calcium contained in cow's milk is relatively useless because it doesn't have sufficient magnesium to allow it all to be fully absorbed and used by the body. In fact, it only has enough magnesium content to allow approximately 11% of what's ingested to be absorbed. It's also interesting to note the nations that produce and consume the largest amounts of dairy foods, are also the nations where the population suffers from the highest levels of osteoporosis. Look at the data relating to this for Holland, the Scandinavian countries, New Zealand, the United States, and Germany. The facts are plain to see, and they're shocking.

Dairy will help to make you fat, and cause bloating. This is because, of the calories derived from fat, whole milk derives about 49%, Cheddar cheese derives about 74%, butter derives 100%. Even 2% fat milk derives about 35%. Therefore, dairy products can easily add hundreds of calories to your diet, simply because they're calorie-dense. This doesn't even take into consideration any of the other issues caused by the fats themselves, or the insulin spikes associated with drinking milk because of the high lactose content of milk. Since it takes roughly ten pounds of milk to produce one pound of cheese, it means that cheese is 10 times as concentrated as milk in terms of what it contains. As for butter, it's about 21 times as dense as milk, so the concentrated content is 21 times richer.

A dairy allergy is one of the most common sources of stomach bloating, and other immune system responses. Furthermore, there are about 12% of the US population who are officially lactose intolerant.

We've already established that lactose is a milk sugar which is comprised of two other forms of sugar, glucose and galactose. We've also established that most adults either lack or produce insufficient quantities of the lactase enzyme which enables them to be broken down. Therefore, without this enzyme, or with not enough of it, lactose is forced to be broken down by bacteria in the lower intestines. During this process, the body's natural waste products combine with the lactose sugars and they ferment. The result of this process is bloating, stomach cramps, and diarrhoea. This directly links into the immune response mechanism which then causes many other dairy allergy related issues.

Dairy has a negative effect on the skin, and it increases the ageing process. Since milk contains lots of sugars, and it also produces a state of acid blood, it naturally causes the skin to wrinkle, and it will often give you acne in the process. This problem is further fuelled by dairy products causing an increase in the production of sebum, which will clog your pores, produce a poor complexion, and aggravate the acne. This situation is made even worse due to the presence of IGF-1, which is one of four growth hormones found in milk. This has the effect of making acne spread, swell, and become highly inflamed. Dairy products have also strong links to aggravating the symptoms of eczema.

In general, dairy products are rich in casein, the milk protein which is linked to causing cancer. This fact alone should be a good enough reason to give up dairy. Milk also contains growth hormones, and the most powerful human growth hormone is identical to the most powerful bovine growth hormone. That same hormone instructs every cell in the human body to grow. Including cancer cells.

There have been many studies conducted about this, and they all conclude the direct link between consuming dairy products and cancer production in humans. Research by Dr T. Colin Campbell even showed that casein, which is 87% of the protein found in milk, promoted ALL the stages of the cancer process. In fact, the link between casein and cancer was so conclusive, that in clinical tests, scientists could literally turn on, and turn off cancer production in rats by simply altering the amount of casein in their diet. Research showed that a diet which comprised of more than 5% of casein turned on cancer production, and diets which comprised of less than 5%, down to zero casein, turned off cancer production.

Dairy makes your whole body weaker and ill. There's now clear scientific evidence, despite what the dairy producers say, the science clearly shows that dairy products are related to diseases and illnesses such as diabetes, joint problems, allergies, heart disease, constipation, asthma, rheumatoid arthritis, lymphoma, and multiple sclerosis.

---

## HELEN WRITES

### Helen's "Lightbulb" Moment About Dairy Foods

*Naturally, for years I have eaten all kinds of dairy products, cheese, yoghurt, milk, etc. However, when I first started training for my Bikini Fitness bodybuilding competitions, I was informed that I would have to give up my beloved dairy foods.*

*Initially, even just the thought of giving up cheese was appalling to me, because I literally put cheese on everything ate! Reluctantly though, I did what my coach told me to do, and gave it all up. Eventually, after a few weeks, the cravings for dairy foods, and especially for cheese, finally stopped.*

*I genuinely thought that I had successfully given up dairy, and I'd also competed in my first competition. With my first competition over, and after meeting veteran coach, Brian Sterling-Vete, who'd advised me to do some independent research into how much protein I really needed, I also realized something else which completely shocked me.*

*During my research into protein and advanced nutrition, I suddenly realized the contradictory and completely confusing information I had been following. Even though I had thought that I had completely given up dairy products as advised, I hadn't. I had never given it a second thought at the time. I suddenly realized that I was still consuming large quantities of dairy products, because whey protein **is** dairy. I was stunned and surprised at myself for not realizing the "obvious" sooner.*

*As soon as I discovered all of this, I switched from whey protein to a vegan-based protein powder, and after a couple of weeks, all the adverse side effects I used to get from the whey protein had stopped. During the transition process though, there was a point when I ran out of my vegan protein powder, and because I still had some whey protein left over, I substituted it for a couple of days.*

*The Sunday prior, I had taken a photo of myself with a completely flat tummy, I was looking and feeling good, prepping for my competition. However, by the following Wednesday, after only two days of consuming whey protein, I seriously looked like I was 20 weeks pregnant!*

*Never again will I use a whey-based protein, and I strongly urge everyone to do the same. Don't get "sold" into the myth of how good whey protein is, because it really isn't. It's just not good for your body.*

*As well as the side-effects I've written about in this book, my own independent research also revealed just how cancerous dairy protein is. I was also completely shocked to*

129

*find out that dairy products help to GIVE you osteoporosis, not prevent it, which is the opposite of everything we're "sold" about dairy products.*

*Dairy products, and dairy-based supplements are sold to an unwitting public as being healthy, yet they'll bring the consumer nothing but allergies, illness, disease, and possibly even death.*

## The Un-Denatured Myth

Since we've been examining the subject of dairy products, and the "supposed" value of whey protein, we may as well examine another aspect of the myth. This is an aspect which is often extolled and exploited by clever marketing. Un-denatured

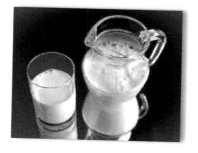

whey protein is becoming popular with bodybuilders. With clever marketing by the supplement manufacturers, at the time of writing, un-denatured whey protein is gaining a mythical status, just like standard whey supplements did before it They're targeting the weaknesses of fitness and bodybuilding enthusiasts who don't really know what it really means. As we mentioned earlier, it has often been said that most bodybuilders are so obsessed that they would eat horse "poop" if a celebrity bodybuilder endorsed it, or if they genuinely thought it might help them to grow a little more muscle or lose some fat. The myth about un-denatured whey is an excellent example of precisely that same phenomena.

To some degree, all whey protein is denatured. Therefore, a good place to start is by establishing exactly what "denatured" means. Denaturing simply means causing "a change in the primary, secondary, or tertiary material, which removes it from its original, and natural state." This includes any process that changes milk from the original way/state that it was in when it exited the cow. For example, skimming the fat from milk is a very common form of denaturing. Denatured protein behaves differently from unaltered protein, and not necessarily in a better way. This is because when protein is denatured, other elements might also become changed in the process. These can include the vitamin content, etc., and in doing so, they may then function less efficiently.

It's illegal to sell raw milk to the public. Therefore, all milk undergoes a process known as pasteurisation. This is a process which was invented by French scientist Louis Pasteur in 1864, when he discovered that heating beer and wine, even slightly, was still enough to kill off most of the bacteria which caused them to turn sour quickly.

For milk, pasteurisation typically means that it has been heated to 72 °C (161 °F) for 16 seconds, and then cooled to 4 °C to ensure that any harmful bacteria are destroyed. This is known as a "high-temperature, short-time" (HTST) pasteurisation process. However, in the United States, the FDA has legalised a process of pasteurisation to heat milk to 63 °C (145 °F) for 30 minutes, which can have an enormous impact on the potency of the "nutrients" it contains.

To summarise, un-denatured whey protein is a form of whey protein that hasn't been altered. Therefore, un-denatured whey protein is more bio-active than pasteurised whey protein. This also means that any increases in its bio-activity will also potentially increase the potency it has in promoting the adverse side effects whey protein typically produces. This also includes making it much more efficient in turning on cancer production, and allergies, in humans.

## The Ketogenic (Keto) Diet

Recently, there's been a lot of renewed interest on the social media platforms, and on certain fitness and bodybuilding forums, about the keto diet. We'll present a few facts about it, express our uncensored opinion, and then leave you to decide for yourself about it.

Ketogenic diet medicine is used primarily to treat epilepsy in children, especially the sort that is difficult to control by other methods. It's a high-fat, low-carbohydrate, and adequate protein diet, which forces the body to burn fat as a primary fuel, instead of carbohydrates.

If there is an extremely low level of carbohydrate in your diet, the liver converts fat into fatty acids and ketone bodies. The body naturally reserves the protein for other uses, and it can only metabolize a certain quantity of protein at any one time. Once that saturation point is reached, excess protein can be converted into energy, which a process called gluconeogenesis. The ketone bodies which are produced when following this type of diet, then pass into the brain to replace glucose as the energy source. It is the elevated level of these ketones in the blood which directly leads to a reduction in the frequency of epileptic seizures.

Fitness people, body shapers, and especially bodybuilders, have found that diets like this are useful fat-loss tools which can even have some favourable health-related benefits. However, for many people, it might seem counterintuitive to eat fat, especially if you're trying to use stored fat for energy to lose fat. However, it doesn't work quite like that. Fat from your diet doesn't produce high levels of insulin response in the body that it would after a meal consisting of high levels of simple carbohydrates. The result is, that the body continues to access stored fat as a source of energy to burn.

Keto-adaptation occurs over a period of weeks when your body becomes accustomed to changing from using carbohydrates as energy, and over to stored fat. The term to be "keto-adapted" simply refers to your body's adaptation to using ketones as its primary energy source.

Since we know that the keto diet will help you to burn more stored body fat, what are the dangers, if any, associated with the diet? To begin with, in the early stages of following a keto diet it's typical to suffer from a certain degree of fatigue and energy loss. This is due to a lower level of blood sugar, and it doesn't usually last too long once the body has become better adapted to the dietary changes. However, many people typically report that they suffer headaches as one of the most obvious side-effects. From an overall health perspective, it should be remembered that ketones are an acid, and therefore, your blood will become more acid from following a keto diet.

Your body is good at responding though, and its quiet adept at buffering some of this acid with calcium. However, since it takes some of this from your bones, it raises the issue of long-term bone density issues being a side effect of following the keto diet. Kidney stones, constipation, gout, nutritional deficiencies, and a plethora of other long-term health issues, including a higher risk of cancer, are also directly related to having highly acidic blood levels because of following the keto diet.

In our opinion, if your long-term health doesn't mean very much to you, then a long-term keto diet might work for you. We believe there are simply too many not-so-nice side-effects related to the keto diet to make it worthwhile. It may be a useful short-term, occasional-use tool, but since we're focussed on overall health, we'd recommend avoiding it, or at the very least only following it very occasionally for brief periods.

## *Alcohol, Health and Body-Fat*

Perhaps surprisingly, research has shown that there are certain health-related benefits to consuming a small quantity of alcohol. I first became aware that there may be certain health-related benefits to consuming a small quantity of alcohol when my Mother became ill with heart disease whilst in her early 90's. During this time, I came to know many senior medical surgeons in England who treated her. Interestingly, they all agreed that consuming small, infrequent quantities of alcohol, was almost certainly better than taking commercial blood-thinning drugs. In their considered opinion, when weighed in the balance, alcohol caused fewer side-effects than drugs, which is something many people in the USA might find shocking.

This is also a great example of what we both love about the practicality, and honesty, found in the not-for-profit British National Health Service. 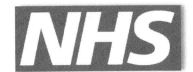 As opposed to the entirely-for-profit US system, where they always want to sell you a drug, a referral, an appliance, or a surgery.

In addition to this, there are also many independent studies which concluded that certain wines are beneficial to health, mostly due to the antioxidants and other macro-nutrients they contain.

While all of this may be true, there are also many people who take this data, and then use it as an excuse to drink a great deal more than the small quantities suggested by some surgeons, and those trained in the medical studies.

Such people conveniently forget that there are also a great many more studies, which have all concluded that excessive alcohol consumption can have a devastating effect on your health, and your bodyweight.

We could droll-on for line-after-line about what alcohol does to the body and brain, but we won't. Instead, we'll get right to the point that most people will be interested in, which is "what effect does alcohol have on body weight, and especially fat loss?" When you consume alcohol, your blood vessels carry it right through your stomach and intestinal tract to your liver.

Once it's in your liver it's then metabolised with an enzyme called dehydrogenase to be converted into acetaldehyde, and after that, it's metabolised into acetate. Once the alcohol has been multi-metabolised

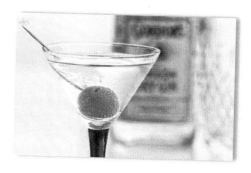

to become acetate, this is where it becomes a problem in terms of fat loss, and weight gain.

One of the main problems is that acetate stops the process of fat oxidation, which in turn means that instead of burning body fat, your body burns the acetate as fuel instead. Only after that's been burned, and depleted, does your body begin burning your stored body fat once again.

Therefore, since you can't easily burn-off the effects of excess alcohol consumption, your body simply accumulates more stored body fat as an energy reserve. In addition to this, alcohol is high in completely worthless calories, with one shot (1.5oz) of vodka (80 proof) containing nearly 100 calories. The bottom line is very simple. The more alcohol you consume, the fatter and unhealthier you will become.

## *Alcohol, Bodybuilding, and Body Shaping*

Even for women, testosterone is very important when it comes to success in bodybuilding and body shaping. We should stress that we're only talking about the levels of testosterone which occur naturally in your body, and NOT about taking additional testosterone to boost your natural capacity for muscles size, shape, and overall athletic performance.

Some clinical studies have shown that when consumed in large quantities, often while binging on alcohol, some men may react by showing a temporary surge in testosterone levels. This brief hormonal jump can partly explain, but certainly not condone, the many well-documented unwarranted drunken sexual advances, and drunken aggression, which can temporarily accompany excess alcohol consumption.

Most of the studies clearly show that in the broader picture, excess alcohol consumption considerably reduces your testosterone levels. Even more alarming is the fact that in some cases, the long-term excessive consumption of alcohol can permanently reduce your normal testosterone levels.

To summarise, the effects of lowered levels of testosterone include:

- Decreased sex drive
- Loss of muscle
- Weight gain due to increased levels of body fat
- Higher blood pressure
- Male breasts (gynecomastia)
- Depression
- Erectile dysfunction
- Heart disease

There is one upside of alcohol consumption for women, which is that it increases oestrogen levels, which in turn can have a positive effect on breast size. Naturally, this is entirely dependent on the individual, and if it occurs, the side-effect is only usually very slight. Therefore, when you balance the numerous negative effects of alcohol, against the positive effects, drinking alcohol in a concerted effort to grow bigger boobs is a non-starter.

## Alcohol and Protein Synthesis

Synthesising protein efficiently is an essential factor in your post-exercise recovery process, and alcohol consumption lowers your protein synthesis efficiency by about 20%. This is because alcohol blocks the absorption of vital nutrients, including potassium, iron, phosphorus, magnesium, and calcium, with the latter having a negative effect on your overall bone density levels.

In addition to this, alcohol also causes dehydration. This means that when your cells aren't flushed to their natural capacity with water, the lack of hydration will impair the muscle building process. One study even revealed that alcohol reduced insulin-like Growth Hormone-1 (or IGF-1) by as much as 40%, which is very significant when you're trying to get into your best shape.

## Hyper-Hydration

The human body is made up of between approximately 60 and 65% water, with your blood holding about 82%, muscle tissue about 72%, and fat holding just 15%. Therefore, it won't come as any surprise to learn that adequate hydration is essential to your overall good health, as well as to muscle building and fat loss.

Unsurprisingly, when you hydrate, the water goes mostly to the places in the body which contain the most water, and thus need to maintain a higher level of

138

hydration. This means that muscle comes before body fat in the water replenishment stakes.

In terms of fat loss, and in helping your body to perform this process more efficiently, you need to ensure that the organs that are essential to this process, are all kept well hydrated.

Ensuring the adequate hydration of both the kidneys and the liver is essential because these two organs play crucial roles in the process of metabolising body fat. If they're already under pressure simply because of lacking proper hydration, then they will be much less efficient at burning body fat.

When it comes to drinking plenty of water each day, there can be a downside. This is when drinking water impacts your sleep due to the constant need to visit the bathroom during the night. It's best to drink most of your daily water intake during the morning and then spread the rest out later in the day in decreasing amounts as you head towards bedtime.

There can always be too much of a good thing though, and the same rule applies when it comes to drinking water. Too much water can cause a condition called hyponatremia, which means that your sodium levels are too low. A sad example of the effects of this condition was felt at Fort Stewart, GA, in the United States in 1999. During basic training, a recruit was hospitalised due to suspected heat exhaustion, which was a misdiagnosis. As a result, the patient was given too much hydration as part of the treatment process. Unfortunately, this excess hydration resulted in the sad death of the recruit in question.

There is a direct relationship to the concentration, and volume, of minerals in your sweat, and the effects which are suffered as a result. These can include muscle cramps, nausea, dizziness and even death. Electrolyte drinks are a good substitute for plain water, especially if you're exercising for longer periods, typically lasting longer than 45 minutes in a single session. Naturally, this isn't a problem for people who follow the ISOfitness™ system of exercise, this is because all workouts are both extremely intense, and extremely brief. However, if you are someone who enjoys other forms of additional physical activity, longer periods of time, then all the factors about hydration must be carefully considered.

## Chapter 4: Genetics, Epigenetics, and "Stuff"

Surprisingly, it now seems that your genetics are no longer a valid excuse as to why you're overweight. Science is slowly eliminating all the excuses that were once thought to be "solid."

We're all blessed with our own unique genetic structure, and there's not much we can do about that. However, we can still positively affect the size and shape of our body, even though it's going to be easier for some people than it is for others. Science has recently proven something which is quite remarkable. This is that your genetic makeup can be affected, and even altered, by external forces. These external forces include whatever it is that you unquestioningly think and believe in, together with the environment you live in.

New research strongly suggests that factors such as environment, and especially your absolute beliefs, together with the resultant mechanisms that are triggered by those beliefs, all play an important role in determining the physical expressions of your genetic code. These effects, and their influences are called "epigenetic." The prefix, "epi" has Greek origins, and it simply means: "upon," "near to," and "in addition."

None of this should come as any surprise to the traditional-thinking members of the medical profession. This is because, the power of "The Placebo Effect" is well known about, well documented, and well accepted. A placebo is typically a simulated, physically inert treatment for a medical condition, or disease, which is intended to deceive the recipient as to its clinically measurable efficacy. The Placebo Effect is still the subject of much scientific research which aims to fully understand the underlying neurobiological mechanisms of the placebo's action in pain relief, immunosuppression, Parkinson's disease, and even depression.

To help try to solve this mystery, scientists have even performed brain imaging on test subjects who have clearly demonstrated that a placebo has had a real, measurable effect on physiological changes in the brain. The Placebo Effect is a pervasive phenomenon which plays an important role in all medical treatments. This is because of the brains perceived, and expected, response to receiving medication. Research has found that the stronger the feelings a person has about the efficacy of the medication, then the more likely it is that the person will experience positive effects and better results. Some studies have clearly shown that there are actual physical changes that occur in a person who completely believes in the effect of something. There is even scientifically documented evidence about physical increases in the production of endorphins in test subjects.

## *Thinking Yourself Strong*

The same effect is true in what someone believes about exercise, and the results they will get from it. There is now clear scientific proof about how the power of your belief can initiate physical changes in your body in relation to exercise. More importantly, your genetics do not necessarily determine your ultimate physical destiny in the way it was previously thought that they did. Therefore, this means that just because your parents may have been overweight, science has now proven that it doesn't necessarily mean that you also must be overweight. The determining factor is whatever your absolute belief and self-image might be, about the size and shape of your body.

The concept that external influences such as your thoughts, environment, exercise, lifestyle, and nutrition can all influence the way your genes express themselves is still new. However, the science of epigenetics is a 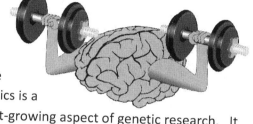 fascinating, and fast-growing aspect of genetic research. It scientifically validates what the great motivational speakers such as Zig Ziglar have been telling everyone for years. This is that the physical expression of "you," will ultimately be determined by whatever you absolutely believe about "you." It also validates what good strength and fitness coaches have also taught for years. This is that whenever you train your body, the quality of the results you get from it, will be directly determined by how you focus your thoughts on the results that you believe you're going to get from the exercise. In other words, you can literally "think" yourself to success in your athletic endeavours, and especially in helping to determine the ultimate size and shape of your body.

Since it's clear that the brain, and what we absolutely believe about something, can have an enormous effect on our physical bodies to a much greater degree than anyone had previously considered. Pioneers in the field of epigenetics, and how the power of our beliefs affect us physically, are making some surprising new discoveries which are having a dramatic impact on the concepts of exercise and muscle growth.

It's becoming increasingly clear that it's vitally important to completely focus the mind on the exercise that is being performed. In addition to this, the same focus and envisioning must be applied to the muscles growing and becoming stronger.

This is bad news for everyone who chooses to listen to music and/or watch TV while exercising. Anything which causes even a slight distraction and loss of concentration will mean that you're never going to get 100% return from your hard work. This concept shouldn't be too surprising, especially since it's the neural pathways in the brain which conduct the stimuli needed to determine the intensely of the contractions within the muscle when it's being exercised.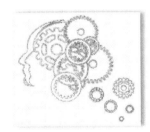

When the neural pathways are increased, the result is that the intensity of the muscular contraction produced also increases, which in turn makes the muscle grow larger and stronger as a result. The increased neural pathways will also lead to the muscular contractions becoming much more controlled, and smooth. It's the same process that eventually allows us to develop extremely refined sporting skills, like those seen in Olympic gymnasts.

These discoveries directly impact how, and when, an isometric contraction exercise should be performed, especially when in conjunction with an isotonic exercise. To derive the maximum benefit from the isometric portion of the exercise, it's always going to be better to do it when you're well rested. To have pre-fatigued your neural pathways with many sets and repetitions of a traditional isotonic exercise, and then to perform an isometric hold on the last repetition, is never going to achieve the best results.

This is because isometric exercise engages almost all the muscle fibres, therefore, it places a much higher demand on your neural pathways and central nervous system. This means that when performing an isometric exercise in combination with an isotonic exercise, the isometric portion should be performed BEFORE the isotonic portion. Alternatively, you can perform the isometric exercise at a separate, dedicated time, at least several hours after performing other types of traditional exercise.

We expect to see some extraordinary breakthroughs announced about the fascinating subject of epigenetics and the power of absolute belief, in the months and years to come. For more information the science of epigenetics, we'd highly recommend the excellent book called "The Biology of Belief," by Bruce H. Lipton PhD. He's the former assistant professor at the University of Wisconsin School of Medicine and a developmental biologist. More recently, Bruce Lipton has become best known for his cutting-edge research into how genes and DNA can be manipulated by a person's absolute beliefs.

### *Base Metabolic Rate (BMR) Explained*

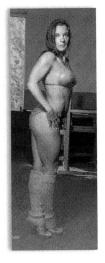

You'll hear a lot about the term "Base Metabolic Rate," or BMR for short, so I'm going to explain what it is now. If you already know what it is, then please forgive this necessary explanation for those who don't, and simply skip this section.

Your metabolism is basically the term for the chemical reactions taking place in the cells of your body which provide the energy to sustain and maintain your life. In simple terms, your BMR is the rate at which your body burns energy to carry out the functions related to maintaining your life. For the average person, this means that about 20% of your overall energy is burned during daily activities. Obviously, this percentage changes if you exercise regularly. It rises according to both the amount of exercise and the intensity of the exercise being performed during your workout sessions.

If 20% of your daily energy is used to just keep you alive, and if you use about 10% of your energy to digest and process the food you eat, this leaves 70% of your energy left-over to be burned during the activities which fill the rest of your day. If you rested and did nothing all day, then you'd still burn a percentage of the remaining potential store of 70% energy which you have in reserve. The rate at which you burn this energy is your Base Metabolic Rate.

A good analogy would be that your BMR is like the amount of fuel your car burns when it's just sitting there, with the engine switched on and ticking-over while you're parked. If the engine is small, which directly compares to a person who isn't carrying much muscle, then even at rest when parked, it won't burn a lot of fuel. This is unlike a larger car engine which will burn more fuel, and which is in direct comparison to a larger person who carries much more muscle.

The more muscle mass you have, the faster your BMR will be. This is a major benefit of exercising and growing more muscle because the natural side-effect is that you will burn more energy as a result. Muscular people will just naturally burn more body fat.

As a person ages, they will gradually lose much of their lean muscle mass, and their BMR will then gradually slow down as part of the process. This is just one of the reasons why it's especially important to exercise regularly throughout your life, no matter what age you are.

It's worth remembering that your body has certain auto-response defence mechanisms to safeguard your life. One of which slows down your BMR rapidly if you crash-diet, and suddenly eat virtually nothing.

This mechanism, which developed over thousands of years of evolution, "believes" that there's a famine. It then causes your body to automatically conserve energy reserves, to help preserve your life until the famine is over. This means that your body will respond to starvation-type diets by dramatically slowing down your weight loss. Crash diets simply don't work, and they aren't healthy either.

## N.E.A.T. - Non-Exercise Activity Thermogenesis

The acronym: N.E.A.T. is becoming increasingly discussed in relation to weight control, body fat, and exercise. The N.E.A.T. acronym stands for Non-Exercise Activity Thermogenesis, and it comes from Dr James Levine's research into how we expend calories. In simple terms means it means: "burning calories through daily life, and not through exercise," and in very simple terms it means that people who are active and move around a lot, burn more calories and tend to be slimmer than people who don't. The people who prefer to sit on their lazy arse and watch TV instead.

There are two basic ways in which we burn calories. One is while we exercise, and the other is through the general activities of daily living. The key question is: "which, if any, is more important to weight loss, and the levels of body fat that we carry?" According to Dr Levine, it's the N.E.A.T. that appears to be far more important for calorie burning than dedicated exercise time. Dr Levine's research also led to the phrase: "Being Active Naturally" becoming more commonly used.

Providing that you're exercising good judgement in your food choices, and in the macros around proper portion control of your food, then in addition to your regular exercise routine, by just being a little more active in everyday life, it will make a huge difference in terms of weight control, and your overall level of body fat.

For example, when we went on location around the U.K. to shoot some pictures and video as part of our

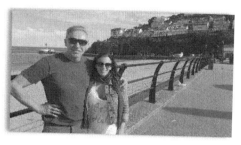

"Fitness on the Move™" workout anywhere concept, we deliberately kept track of how many steps we took, and how active we were each day. Prior to the trip, we logged an average of between 5,000 and 10,000 steps per day, depending upon what we were doing business-wise or socially. From the day we landed in London, and then travelled to Manchester, and onward around the North West, our daily step count jumped up markedly. When we were on location in both Cornwall and Cumbria, the numbers increased dramatically. In Cornwall, our daily step counts never dropped below 18,000, except for the day we arrived, and the day we left. During the entire time we were there it averaged in the 18,000 to 20,000 step range, with occasional spikes to between 20,000 and 25,000 when we were hiking up and down the steep ocean cliffs between the tiny fishing villages on the Cornish coastal path. All this activity resulted in our N.E.A.T. increasing dramatically, and it left plenty of room for portion-controlled treats such as good old British fish and chips while managing to easily maintain our desired levels of body fat and overall weight.

In our opinion, N.E.A.T. alone isn't the great panacea when it comes to losing weight and staying slim. After all, when people are stressed and mentally fatigued because of a tough workday, then it's not always easy to opt for the most sensible food choices, nor is it likely that you're going to want to go out and do something active to increase your daily movement factor. However, N.E.A.T. is certainly something to be factored into your overall lifestyle because it really does make a significant difference to your overall appearance and fitness levels.

## *Thermodynamics*

Thermodynamics is the science of heat and temperature, and their relation to energy. When it comes to weight loss and burning more body fat, the same rules of science apply. This means that by following a few simple rules of common-sense thermodynamics, it will equal a leaner "you" as a result.

We all know, or at least we should all know, that it takes energy to maintain your body temperature at 98.6 degrees Fahrenheit. This energy consumption is part of your overall Base Metabolic Rate. This means that if you create a cooler environment for your body, it will automatically burn more stored body fat as the energy needed to protect itself and maintain a stable core temperature.

Simple tricks to help burn more calories with little or no extra effort are based around keeping you cooler, for longer. Things such as: never using an electric blanket, keeping your central heating at home set at a slightly lower-than-comfortable temperature, wearing fewer clothes, avoiding wearing hats since massive amounts of your body heat escapes through your head, avoiding sauna baths in lieu of cooler showers etc. These simple things will all add up to making your body burn more calories to maintain your protected core temperature.

However, never cool yourself to dangerously low levels, possibly even to the hypothermia stage. The adjustments in lifestyle/temperature control that we mentioned are all very slight. They absolutely do not include things like sitting on blocks of ice or forcing yourself to be outdoors in sub-zero temperatures while only wearing your superhero underwear.

If incorporated and applied sensibly, correctly, and in a balanced proportion, then employing the use of thermodynamic cheating methods can be an easy way to help you maintain a leaner, and healthier body weight.

## *Spot Reduction*

When people who are new to the world of fitness, body shaping, and bodybuilding, they often ask initially about how they can reduce the size of their stomach, or another particularly flabby and out of shape part of their body. This is technically called "spot reduction," and it's the supposed ability to affect only 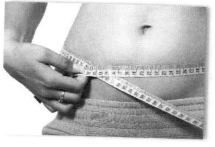 the levels of excess body fat you carry in specific places on the body, such as around your waistline.

We may as well burst your bubble right now. Natural spot reduction of body fat does not work. It's a myth that is often generated, and then perpetuated, by the manufacturers of cosmetic treatments, creams, wraps, and general "miracle" creams. Basically, it's all complete nonsense designed to appeal to lazy people.

The facts are very simple, to change the size and shape of your body, to lose fat, to achieve a flat stomach, or to get any other part of you into better shape, then it still all comes down to a few basic rules. it requires a combination of healthy low-calorie eating, making better food choices, increasing your Base Metabolic Rate, taking regular exercise, and burning a combination of visceral fat, subcutaneous fat, and intramuscular fat. In addition to this, you also need to eliminate any kind of single-session over-eating, and drinking too much liquid, especially alcohol. These negative processes will physically stretch the stomach, which certainly won't help matters, and it will also contribute to the classic "beer-belly" effect.

It's worth remembering that performing stomach exercises, such as trunk curls, AKA: sit-ups alone isn't the best way to reduce your waist size. Of course, they're an excellent way of toning the stomach muscles, but they're not a great calorie burner, or Base Metabolic Rate stimulator. You'll reduce your waist size much more rapidly by burning more stored body fat, which will be achieved more efficiently by performing higher calorie-burning exercises such as squats, running, or chin-ups. These will also provide a greater stimulus to increase your BMR. Therefore, when you perform trunk curls, it may feel as though you're directly attacking the problem area to help flatten your stomach, however, they won't. Stick to the higher calorie-burning exercises instead.

153

## A "Best Way" To Lose Body Fat?

The best way to lose body fat and maintain muscle mass is always going to be to reduce your calorie intake to just a fraction below the point where you eat just enough to maintain your bodyweight. At the same time increasing your Base Metabolic Rate through high intense resistance-based exercise.

If fat loss is your overall goal, then you're best using Short Burst Training (SBT) / High-Intensity Interval Training (HIIT) routines. This is because these systems have greater long-term post-exercise fat burning effects than "traditional" aerobic exercises. These are the real names for some of the "fancy-schmancy" hyped-up names used to describe exercise systems are sold in many of the TV infomercials. Save your money, put your brain into gear, do some proper research, and you'll get some great results without paying a small fortune for it.

## Walking Vs Running as a Fat Burner

Walking and running are both an excellent way to get fitter, burn calories, tone up, and promote weight loss.

However, there are different and distinct benefits to each. Running burns more calories than walking does. However, walking burns more fat than running 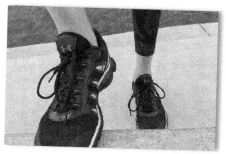 does. So, it's a trade-off, especially since walking more will increase your N.E.A.T. factor.

When exercising at a lower intensity, fat is being used as the body's primary fuel. When you shift-gears and increase the pace from walking to running, then your body burns more carbohydrates as fuel. It doesn't really matter too much if you're burning body fat as the primary fuel, or if you're just burning carbohydrate as the primary fuel. What is important is that you burn the most calories possible during your exercise session and stimulate a long-term increase in your Base Metabolic Rate. Therefore, even though walking may burn more stored fat as fuel, running will still burn more overall calories.

Another important factor to consider when looking at the differences between walking and running are the risks of injury from each. Running carries more risk of injury than walking, so the choice is yours.

### Cardio Vs Resistance Training as a Fat Burner

At a basic level, cardiovascular training usually burns more calories than weight training. However, for serious calorie burning, High-Intensity Interval Training (HIIT) will have a greater fat burning effect than performing traditional cardiovascular exercises alone.

High-Intensity Interval Training will ensure that more overall calories are burned during the exercise period itself. In addition, the enhanced calorie-burning effect generated by stimulating your Base Metabolic Rate will continue through the following 24-hour post-exercise recovery period.

The best overall types of workout that deliver the fastest results when it comes to fat loss are SBT, AKA Short

Burst Training, and HIT, AKA High-Intensity Training, with the latter referring to purely high-intensity weight training. The best regimen would probably include, and combine, High-Intensity Interval Training to maximise the calories burned, together with a high-intensity weight training routine to stimulate the maximum muscle gains. Keep your workouts short, focussed, and intense.

## *Acronyms, Acronyms, Acronyms*

Acronyms seem to be everywhere in our daily life and business, and the same is true in the world of exercise science, or perhaps even more so. When you enter the world of exercise you'll immediately notice that many confusing acronyms are used which include:

- ▲ SBT which is the acronym for Short Burst Training.
- ▲ HIT which is the acronym for High-Intensity Training.
- ▲ HIIT which is the acronym for High-Intensity Interval Training.
- ▲ HIRT which is the acronym for High-Intensity Resistance Training.
- ▲ AIT which is the acronym for Aerobic Interval Training.

There are a great many more, and we won't bore you with a longer list than is absolutelyu necessary for us to make our point. At the top of the list, you'll notice the following acronyms: SBT, HIT and HIIT.

These are the ones that seem to cause those who are new to exercise the most confusion. Even though we briefly touched on SBT and HIIT in the previous section, we'll explain them in a little more depth.

For most people who simply want to exercise and who aren't serious sports people or professional athletes, then SBT and HIIT are so similar that they're essentially the same thing.

The principles behind SBT and HIIT are basically variants of circuit training. They employ a series of high-intensity, short-duration exercises interspersed with brief periods of lower-intensity exercises. The intent is to train at the highest intensity possible for bursts of between 30 and 60 seconds, dependent upon the intensity employed.

The anaerobic (without air) burst of higher intensity exercise is followed by a recovery period, which employs lower intensity cardio exercises. The sequence is then repeated for the entire duration of the workout session. One of the most basic, and common workouts, in this category would be 30 to 45 seconds of intense sprinting, which is alternated with periods of between 15 and 30 seconds of jogging or walking, depending upon the capability of the person exercising.

People might more commonly refer to HIIT being an exercise session which starts with a warm-up period and then leads into a single high-intensity exercise period, followed by a cool-down period to conclude the workout. H.I.T. is a form of resistance training performed at high intensity yet in short duration. It was made popular by the inventor of Nautilus, Arthur Jones, in the 1970s and it advocates performing high-quality repetitions to the point of momentary muscular failure.

The objective is to engage the maximum number of muscle fibres during each exercise, within the framework of a traditional resistance training environment. In following these methods, it's possible to grow both muscle size and strength more efficiently than through traditional, lower intensity resistance training sessions.

H.I.T. will ensure that both the heart rate and metabolism become significantly elevated. In addition, research has found that H.I.T. is more efficient at burning body fat than traditional, lower intensity resistance training. The high-intensity exercises are performed at near maximum physical capacity, which is directly reflected in the short duration of the exercise period itself. The harder and more intensely you exercise, then the shorter the time that you're physically able to perform that exercise.

## Stress, More Stress, "Stuff," and Muscle Growth

Many factors can affect muscle growth, including sex, age, sleep, and nutrition. An adequate supply of amino acids in your diet is essential to muscle growth, together with the presence of enough testosterone in your body. As we know, testosterone is one of the body's major growth hormones, and since men naturally have more of this hormone than women, it's also why men find it easier to grow larger muscles than women. Taking additional testosterone 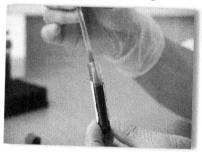 will increase your muscle building results. It also involves some very serious risks to your health in both the short-term, and long-term. The use of testosterone supplements, anabolic steroids, and other performance-enhancing drugs are not recommended. I have direct experience in how the use of products like testosterone, and anabolic steroids has killed several of my close friends over the years. All these people were in amazing shape, they were multi-contest-winners, strong, muscular, and great overall athletes. One of my friends who foolishly used anabolic steroids, and died as a result, was a multi-world champion.

Most "gym rats" fall into the "It'll never happen to me" brigade. They foolishly believe that they are somehow different, and therefore immune to the terrible side-effects of these things. These drugs do not differentiate between world champions and the ordinary person who joins a gym to grow a little more muscle. Use of these products will eventually weaken, debilitate and eventually kill those who take them. If someone still decides to take additional testosterone, or anabolic steroids, even after thoroughly researching the negative effects they will have on the body, then in our opinion, they deserve zero sympathy in the years to come when they have deliberately wrecked their body.

It's worth remembering this when you see high-level champion bodybuilders of both sexes advertising and promoting food supplements, vitamins, amino acids, and protein supplements in bodybuilding and fitness magazines, these people almost certainly use anabolic steroids, unless they are open drug-free competitors. Does anyone seriously think for one minute that they got into the shape they needed to win the highest level of professional bodybuilding contests naturally, and by simply taking the supplements they're advertising? If anyone thinks that they do, then they're living in their very own "Area 51 – Dreamland." As someone who was one part of the team who were the chief sponsors and producers of the N.A.B.B.A. Mr. and Miss Universe contests for 5 years, and who was also a senior consultant to the sports nutrition company which backed it, I can tell you straight that it doesn't happen any other way.

On a slightly lighter note, other things which can adversely affect muscle growth and good health include, vertebral subluxation, lack of quality sleep, and poor nutrition. All these things can negatively affect your progress towards losing weight and getting into better overall shape. Therefore, get any issues you might have in any, or all, of those areas, corrected as soon as possible so you can be set free to make the best progress possible.

Stress can also have an adverse effect on muscle growth, and especially on your levels of body fat. When you're stressed, your body produces a stress hormone called Cortisol, and this decreases amino acid absorption by muscle tissue, which in turn inhibits protein synthesis and muscle growth.

In addition to this, chronic stress can be directly linked to an increase in your appetite and the associated stress-induced weight gain. This is because the ancient protection mechanisms built into your body and brain, still haven't progressed much beyond the Stone Age. Your body's base-response and protection mechanisms don't recognise much difference between the stress caused by petty problems at work in your office and being chased by an enormous sabre-toothed tiger.

The perceived "threat" that your body registers triggers a series of mechanisms, which then releases both cortisol and adrenaline to give you an instant, but short burst of energy. The Cortisol and Adrenaline in your system will initially cause a temporary decrease in appetite. Once the perceived "threat" has subsided, the Cortisol then causes an **increase** in your appetite. This is because your body wants to replenish the energy it used while you were stressed and to store more reserves of energy just in case you have more similar stress in the future.

To make matters even worse, the first fuel that your body wants to burn during a crisis is sugar. people who are under stress often crave large quantities of carbohydrates. The stress signals that your body produces will trigger your body to store more visceral fat, usually in your midsection area. Any kind of stress, including the stress to the CNS, or Central Nervous System, caused by over-training, can have a serious negative effect on your overall muscle building and fitness gaining progress.

The best way to prevent this is to only perform brief, high-intensity workouts, to always allow yourself a proper recovery period between workouts, to get plenty of quality sleep, and to ensure that you always have good nutrition. If possible, you should always try to keep your stresses to a minimum. Even though this is sometimes easier said than done in daily life, it's still very important to at least try and not allow comparatively unimportant things get to you.

## Somatotyping

Body somatotype is also a significant factor in what you might expect your overall progress to be, as well as your overall maximum potential. It's a category to which people are assigned according to the extent their bodily physique conforms to a basic type. In physiology, the different classifications of human body types are broken down by their basic component tissue types. There are three physical somatotypes which are: Endomorphic, Mesomorph, and Ectomorph.

The pure Endomorphic body is characterised by having:

△ A wide waist
△ Larger bones
△ Otherwise known as being fat

The pure Mesomorph body is characterised by having:

△ Wide shoulders
△ Narrow waist
△ Medium to large bone structure
△ Low body fat
△ Otherwise known as being muscular

The pure Ectomorph body is characterised by having:

△ A slim chest
△ Longer limbs
△ Leaner muscles
△ Low fat
△ Otherwise known as being slim

162

This system of classification was developed in the 1940s, by William Sheldon, who was a noted American psychologist. His system categorised the listed body types according to a scale from 1 to 7. Using this scale, a pure Endomorphic body would be categorised as being 7-1-1, with a pure Mesomorph body being 1-7-1, and the pure Ectomorph body being 1-1-7. The somatotype of every person is expressed as three numbers in succession. As an example, to estimate that the somatotype of, Arnold Schwarzenegger, who's arguably the greatest bodybuilder who ever lived, would be approximately 2-6-2 on the Sheldon scale.

Each person's original genetics determines their individual somatotype, and it also determines what many of their physical strengths and weaknesses are, as well as their peak physical limitations in terms of their overall objectives. This doesn't take into consideration the epigenetic factors, which can also have an enormous effect. Even someone who is a pure Endomorph, someone who is prone to carrying excess fat and who may never be able to compete as a top physique, strength, or gymnastics contender, can still make excellent progress. It is very rare to find that someone falls completely into only one category. Almost everyone falls into a combination of the three categories.

Whilst on this topic, and as a sort of footnote, please don't try to "sell" yourself, or anyone else for that matter, on the pathetic excuse that you have "big bones," and that's why you're overweight. That's complete rubbish because there's no such thing. You may as well blame the tooth fairy for your excess weight. Saying things like this just means that you've found yet another way of making yourself appear to be extremely stupid.

## *Different Types of Muscle Fibre*

The voluntary muscles of the body, which are the ones you exercise to strengthen and get bigger, are composed of different types of fibres, and each type has different properties. The three basic types are as follows:

- ▲ Slow twitch fibres are red in colour because of their high oxygen saturation level and are excellent to support endurance. These fibres are slightly smaller in size than the other fibres, and they usually support your body's structural alignment and overall support structure due to their endurance-supporting qualities.
- ▲ Fast twitch fibres are white in colour due to their comparatively poor oxygen saturation level, and they're excellent for strength and explosive power. These fibres are bigger than slow twitch, intermediate twitch type 2b fibres. They suffer fatigue more rapidly than slow twitch fibres which is why they're not used to support the skeletal structure, and they're mostly found in the large muscles of the legs, chest and arms. These are the fibres predominantly targeted when developing muscular size and strength.
- ▲ Intermediate twitch, or type 2B fibres, which are grey in colour due to their intermediate level of oxygen saturation and are excellent for recruitment in supporting muscle endurance and power.

164

During a set of traditional resistance training of between 8 and 12 repetitions, there is only a partial engagement of each type of muscle fibre taking place.

At the beginning of a repetition, which is almost always at a biomechanically disadvantaged position, type 2 muscle fibres are usually engaged first.  After the first repetition, other factors then come into play, together with the other types of fibre becoming either more or less, engaged during the entire course of the set.

Traditional resistance training doesn't engage any of the different muscle fibre types very efficiently, or for very long.  This is also one of the reasons why traditional resistance training requires that so many arbitrary sets and repetitions to be performed.  This is to get closer to what might be a reasonable level of muscle fibre engagement during an exercise.

Coaches and everyone else who exercises, will typically devise a workout which involves what at best might be an educated guess as to the ideal number of repetitions and sets to be performed, and at worst something that doesn't even get close.

We all know that professional athletes who perform resistance training, are typically closely monitored by knowledgeable and highly qualified sports coaches who usually have a plethora of scientific testing and measuring equipment to hand. This means that they'll be able to both devise a routine and then closely monitor the athlete, so they can more accurately determine exactly what's needed to achieve the desired goal.

For the average person who exercises regularly, where is the science is in performing an arbitrary number of repetitions and sets of each exercise? The answer to that question is easy. There is no science. It's all guesswork. Even after all the years of research, countless books being written, speciality magazines galore, and a myriad of online resources, one thing is constant. This is that the most carefully planned workout regimens devised by people who don't have access to all the high-level testing and measuring equipment, will still all be based on performing an arbitrary recommendation of the number of repetitions for each exercise, and an arbitrary number of sets as well.

In addition, it's highly likely that the arbitrary recommendations made in this respect by both coaches, and practitioners of exercise alike, will be often be based upon little more an article in a fitness magazine, or maybe an online blog. This is as scientific as it generally gets for most people in gyms today.

## Breathing

There may be some people who are tempted to hold their breath at times while performing exercises. This is, of course, a completely stupid thing to do. Unless you're swimming underwater, escaping from a fire, or doing something similar that makes it essential that you hold your breath, then it really isn't a smart thing to do. It seems there are a lot of stupid people in the world who need to be told even the most obvious of things. Therefore, since I've no idea who will read this book, the obvious thing is written here in bold capital letters: **NEVER HOLD YOUR BREATH WHILE PERFORMING ISOMETRICS, OR ANY OTHER KIND OF EXERCISE!** For those intelligent people who are reading this book, please forgive me having to state the obvious in such a way.

When exercising, always breathe naturally, and fully, in and out always. For example, when performing an isometric exercise, we believe that the best way to breathe, and accurately count the number of seconds that each isometric exercise position is held for, is by counting the number of full, deep breaths - in and out - that are taken while performing the exercise. This will naturally be at the rate of approximately one second per complete breath in and out. Employing this technique makes it easy to keep track of how long you perform each exercise for. More importantly, it'll help to ensure that you don't count the seconds too quickly while performing each exercise, and you'll also be sure to get plenty of good air to help oxygenate the blood. It's easy to "cheat" by breathing too quickly, or too shallow. This will typically cause you to count the number of seconds for each exercise too quickly. We'd also recommend that you aim to perform a 10 to 12-second isometric hold. This will almost certainly ensure that you always reach the required 7-second marker without cheating.

For isotonic exercises, the generally accepted best method of breathing is to always inhale on the easier part of each repetition, and exhale on the hard part. Taking the barbell curl as an example, one would breathe in as the weight is lowered, and out as the weight is raised. Naturally, there will always be certain exceptions to this rule, however, for the most part, it can be applied to almost all exercises.

## Getting to Grips

It's essential to always form a strong and stable line of biomechanical progression when performing any exercise, including both isometrics and traditional resistance training. This is because, without a stable line of biomechanical progression, 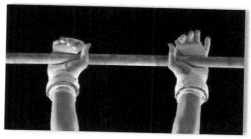 you're always going to be more susceptible to creating weak spots, injuries, and even create conditions which will haunt you in the future, such as tennis elbow.

We're appalled to see how many people in fitness clubs perform exercises such as the bench press. For some unknown reason, some people feel compelled to balance the bar in the palms of an almost open hand, instead of gripping the bar properly. Maybe these people think that it's somehow "cool" for them to exercise this way and that it sends a message to others watching that they're somehow "experienced" at exercising that they can do it in a cool style.

The bad news for anyone who does this is that it's not cool, it's stupid. If they know what to look for, the only message that it sends out to others who watch is that

168

you're not clever enough to understand biomechanics and potential dangers of what you're doing. Using this method, you're helping to create potentially niggling injuries and other issues which will interfere with your overall progress.

A stable line of biomechanical progression begins with a correctly executed and positioned grip. In taking a firm grip this way, you can begin to form a chain of progression and stability, that can then be continued through other correctly aligned joints and limbs while you perform the exercise in good style. The same is true in when it comes to isometric exercises. It begins with a stable line of biomechanical progression, starting with either a properly clenched hand or fist, and then continuing that line of stability through correctly aligned joints and limbs to perform the isometric contraction hold.

This is just one reason why we recommend, and endorse, the excellent Iso-Bow®. This clever little device makes this whole process of forming a strong biomechanical chain, much easier. It has well-designed and comfortable non-slip hand grips, which allow you to create a stable line of biomechanical progression in every exercise.

## *Prevent Injuries and Knotted Muscles*

The secret to success in any sport, and any form of resistance/strength training is to maintain an injury-free status throughout your training year/cycle. This includes remaining "knot-free" and flexible, which is especially important when you perform any high-intensity exercise. If you have a knotted muscle of any sort, it will certainly make itself known during your workout.

The pain signals that are produced because of a serious injury, and even by something as simple as a knotted muscle, is a signal to your brain that there is something wrong. Safety should always come first. The moment you experience any sort of pain you must stop what you're doing, rest, seek medical advice/treatment, possibly apply ice, compression, elevate, and generally give your body time to fully recover.

The golden rule is that you should always let your doctor decide what's best for you. To do otherwise is foolishness. If you do not allow any injury time to heal, then every time you exercise while you have the injury, you will simply be injuring yourself even more, building up scar tissue, and possibly setting yourself on course to have a life-long weakness from the long-term injury.

Today, social media is full of fools who make ridiculous posts about "I've seriously injured my back/elbow/shoulder/whatever, and despite the pain and suffering, I'm enduring it. I'm just sucking it up and training as normal..." I've seen many posts like this, some of which have been made by bodybuilder friends of my wife. Even more amazingly, some of these postings have been made by people who hold an instructor qualification certificate, one which allows them to teach people about fitness and strength. This makes me deeply concerned. If this is their approach and is indicative of their level of intelligence, what does it say about the quality of the "apparently" nationally accepted qualifications they hold to teach exercise. The bad news for people who boast about training through the pain of an injury is that it doesn't make them appear to be more dedicated, tougher, hard-core, or special. Instead, in the eyes of real professionals, and anyone else with even a modicum of common sense, it only makes these people appear to be extremely stupid.

Perhaps the most common form of "injury" is the knotted muscle. Even though this might be comparatively minor when compared to other kinds of common sports-related injuries, it still needs to be treated quickly and effectively. However, the first question we need to answer is: "What exactly is a knotted muscle?"

A knotted muscle is a common term for what is technically known as a myofascial trigger point. The word myofascial is a composite, with "myo" referring to the muscle, and "fascial" referring to the thin, strong, and elastic type of connective tissue surrounding the muscle. The knotted sensation is the point where the muscle has become compressed or constricted in some way, which then generates pain. The pain can be anything from a constant dull ache, a sharp pain when a muscle or limb is moved in a specific way, or it can be a constant sharp pain.

Technically, there are still no definitive answers as to why a knotted muscle forms, and then persists. Instead, there are still only several interesting theories. These range from it being the result of old injuries, micro-trauma – which in terms of muscle tissue is the micro-tearing of muscle fibres, a problem with the sheathing which surrounds the muscle, and dehydration which may help muscle fibres to adhere to each other. There is even a theory if the amount of connective tissue is excessive, then it may contribute to the formation of knots. Scar tissue another suspected cause, because it is composed of a collagen fibrous material that is not very flexible. The problem with scar tissue is that once scar tissue has been created it can adhere to muscle fibres. This adhesion impedes or prevents the muscle fibres from moving smoothly across other uninjured/normal muscle fibre and connective tissue. The result is a loss of flexibility, and often pain.

Interestingly, when muscle tissue from a persistent knot has been removed and analysed, certain anomalies have been found in the protein within the tissue itself.

Whatever the reason, something or a combination of things triggers a reaction which causes a muscular spasm/involuntary and prolonged contraction. This somehow causes a muscle to remain in a state of constant activity, instead of the muscle being able to relax into passive mode. The result of all this is the feeling of tightness in a specific area of the muscle, and lo and behold: you have a "knotted" muscle.

There is still no universally accepted treatment to cure a knotted muscle, instead, the focus is more about effectively managing the condition. Treatments commonly used include ice/hot packs, ultrasound, electrical stimulation, and deep massage. However, two new forms of electrical-based treatment have become available in treatment devices known as the Myopulse, and Acuscope. These versatile instruments have proven to be successful in treating many forms of injuries, and dramatically reducing recovery times. They have also been proven effective in the elimination of scar tissue. Although these instruments are still being tested, the results so far achieved indicate that a significant breakthrough has been made in how sports injuries are treated.

They basically function by sending a microelectronic signal through an injured section of the body. The computer then measures the impedance of the tissue which it passes through. If an anomaly is detected in the electrical impedance of the cells, because of an injury and/or scar tissue. The instruments then send other signals through the tissue, which then try to correct the impedance. In doing so, they either permanently heal the injury, or they dramatically reduce/eliminate the scar tissue. These instruments seem set to revolutionise sports medicine. I'm extremely encouraged, and after reading about some of the science data myself, together with many of the other test results which have yet to be made public, I've already contacted the development team so that I can learn much more about them professionally.

For the immediate future though, professional sports massage still seems to be one of the most effective, and easiest, of the traditional ways to treat a knotted muscle. From my personal experience of having a seriously knotted muscle treated many years ago, massage certainly seems to increase blood flow, increase the flexibility of stubborn scar tissue, and it will generally help the muscle fibres move more smoothly across each other. The important thing to remember is that if for whatever reason you ever find yourself developing a knotted muscle or any other kind of injury, then always stop whatever you are doing right away, and immediately consult your physician. Always let your doctor decide what is best for you, it is that simple.

## Misnomers and More "Stuff"

If you're going to exercise, then it makes complete sense to only use the most effective and efficient systems, to get the best results as quickly as possible. There's simply no point in wasting time by performing less-effective exercises. Many women are seem unduly disturbed at the thought of "shaping" their body by toning and building their muscles. We've no idea what these women think happens when they shape up, but since we've already established that it's impossible to flex fat, then the only solution is to flex some muscle.

Even more ridiculous, are the women who believe that if they exercise with weights or against a resistance, then they'll suddenly sprout huge muscles. This is, of course, an utterly stupid belief because it simply doesn't happen. We suspect that it's part of the common "plexcuse mechanism," which some people rely on to try and explain away why they're not in good shape, and why don't exercise. Women who think this way need somehow navigate themselves into the real world. In our opinion, they don't consider that even a little muscle on a woman, is often enough to create a well-trained muscular backside and thighs, which is always going to be far sexier than if she has an arse which looks more like it was composed of two Japanese Sumo wrestlers in a sack who are trying to escape.

In respect to muscle building, most women simply don't have enough testosterone to build very large muscles. However, they do have more than enough testosterone to effectively shape their body by toning their muscles. Most women can easily stimulate and grow enough muscle to create an aesthetically pleasing body in a very short time. In fact, with regular training, then many women can build high-performance athletic bodies without too much effort. Admittedly, there are some women who do have enough testosterone to build large muscles, which is also great and it's a thing to be admired if they can. However, this is rare. Some women even resort to taking supplemental testosterone, and anabolic steroids, in their quest to build muscle and increase their athletic performance. We are certainly not suggesting that all women bodybuilders do this. When women are carrying almost as much muscle as a man, then most often, they are using drugs. To all the ladies who do this, we all know what you're doing, so please just be open about it and admit it.

## HELEN WRITES

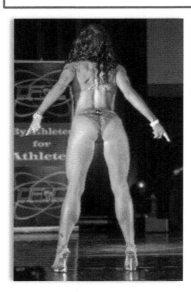

*I admit that I was precisely this type of woman. I was the typical sort of woman who liked to "extend" to the world that I was happy with my body just the way it was, even though I was technically obese. I didn't want to lift weights because I didn't want "MANLY" muscles. Once I saw my twin sister lose the weight and build*

175

*muscle, I must admit, I was a bit surprised at how incredibly sexy she looked with her muscular arms. In no way did it make her manly. She looked sexier and more feminine that I had ever seen.*

Men aren't much different in the "pathetic excuses stakes." Men just use different excuses, and they are equally stupid ones. One of the most common flaws men suffer from is that they usually exercise their ego, instead of exercising their body. They typically do this by trying to always lift *as* much weight as possible, instead of trying to exercise properly with a lighter weight to engage as many muscle fibres as possible. Many men simply don't understand that there's a huge difference between exercising their ego and exercising the muscles. The former makes them feel better for a few moments, while the latter makes them feel, look, and perform better for a long time afterwards. Lifting as much weight as possible in appalling style does absolutely nothing to engage the muscles they're

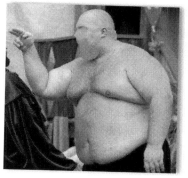

supposed to be targeting. Instead, they're just increasing the risk of injuring themselves and making themselves appear silly in the process.

Oh, by the way, here's some bad news guys... If you can't clearly see your abdominal muscles, AKA: your "6-pack," or at least see them in some reasonable degree of clarity, then you're just one thing: FAT. The clarity of a man's 6-pack, or lack of it, is one of the best indicators as to the amount of body fat he's carrying. The bad news is that it's not hard to identify if a person is fat. There's some other bad news for guys too. Despite what some guys like to think of themselves as being, there's just no such thing as "beefy," "chunky," or "hunky." Those are typically just alternative words meaning that you're big and fat.

Whilst on the general subject of exercise, physique, diet, and getting into shape, we feel compelled to briefly touch upon the subject of cosmetic surgery. This is because "exercise-laziness" literally knows no bounds, and many women, together with a growing number of men too, would even foolishly prefer to rely entirely on having cosmetic surgery in their quest to get into better shape and lose weight. We're completely against people who turn to cosmetic surgery as a first option. These people are just being lazy, excuse-driven, and they also lack enough willpower to modify their diet and do some basic exercises.

People need help to learn how to say "no, I've had enough food." The bad news is that even after they've resorted to having a gastric band fitted, they'll almost always eventually continue to overeat because the real cause of the problem still hasn't been addressed.

The same goes for people who opt for liposuction as a solution to the problem of excess body weight. Having liposuction simply won't work unless it is used in conjunction with lifestyle changes to tackle the cause of the issue. There's just no escaping the fact that for liposuction to be successful long-term, people will always need to modify their diet and take regular exercise. If these changes don't take place, then after having liposuction, it is almost certain that excess body fat will eventually be regained. Very soon, the entire process will need to be repeated. This is the opposite of what we believe liposuction should be used for. We believe that liposuction is an excellent tool, but it's only a tool and not an overall solution. This is because when used as a tool in conjunction with diet and exercise, it can deliver some excellent long-term results. It can deliver results that can add outstanding finishing touches to a well-sculpted body.

In our opinion, we find the most laughable aspect of cosmetic surgery, to be men who have implants to give the appearance of having a more muscular body. Some men resort to surgery to give them the illusion of having biceps, pectoral, and other muscles. Resorting to cosmetic implants to give the illusion of having muscle is, in our opinion, pathetic. These people are too bone-idle, weak-willed, and lazy to build real muscle through exercise. More importantly, what's the point of only appearing to have well-developed muscles? Someone who only appears to have well-developed muscles through implants isn't going to be physically strong, athletic, and fit. They're only ever going to be a proverbial "paper tiger."

Using a car as an analogy, they'll have the exterior of a supercar like an Aston Martin DB9, however, they'll have the physical performance of only a tiny economy vehicle. The exterior image and the physical performance will be two completely contradictory things. Even worse, what do they think will happen if they ever eventually strike-up a serious relationship? What happens then? What happens when the big moment finally comes along, and when your potential life-partner sees them for what they really are.  Physically weak, egocentric, and emotionally impaired – what a catch.

Muscle implants are only useful to counter the physical effects of serious diseases, and physical trauma which has damaged muscle or caused all or part of it to be removed.  These are legitimate and excellent reasons to have muscle implants, as opposed to the cosmetic bodybuilder who is an unfunny caricature of laziness.  There are also completely legitimate reasons why people might opt for cosmetic surgery, such as breast augmentation, liposuction, and/or a tummy tuck, especially after having children.  Giving birth to children can completely change a woman's size, shape, stretched skin, and overall appearance.  Therefore, when used in conjunction with proper diet and exercise, some highly worthwhile procedures can be performed for entirely the right reasons.

## *Brace Yourself*

Knee and elbow braces, support sleeves, compression supports, and weight lifting belts won't cure an issue, they'll only offer some relief.  More importantly, if you wear these things long-term, they'll only serve to make you progressively weaker and less able to be physically active.  This is because since they physically support muscles, joints, ligaments and tendons, they aren't being physically challenged and stimulated.

Without physical stimulation and challenge, your muscles, joints, ligaments and tendons won't get any stronger.  Instead, they'll progressively weaken until you need to increasingly rely on artificial support mechanisms instead of the muscles, joints, ligaments and tendons you need to keep you physically active and strong.

The manufacturers of these devices don't really care if this happens, and why should they? This is because they'll eventually sell you more of their products as you become gradually weaker as time passes. These devices are only a rehabilitation tool, and when used as such, they're excellent. However, they're **ONLY** a rehabilitation tool, and **NOT** a long-term solution.

### On Balance...

I wasn't sure how else to put this, so I'll be blunt as usual. Do not weigh yourself every day. If you do this already, then you're wasting your time, and you're also creating self-doubt and negativity issues as part of your rollercoaster experience. Your body fluid levels are always going to fluctuate daily, and throughout the course of each day. Therefore, to weigh yourself every day, or even several times each day, is a completely pointless waste of time.

It's important to remember that muscle is much denser than fat. Your body weight doesn't necessarily determine your overall levels of stored body fat. A much better indicator for both men and women is what you look like in a mirror. For example, if your abdominal muscles are starting to show a little more, if they're slightly emerging, then it's a good thing. In our opinion, this is a much better body composition indicator than weighing yourself daily.

## Chapter 5: Body Basics

Body shaping is very like bodybuilding, in that you change the size, shape, and overall composition of your body by means of exercise and sensible nutrition. The result is a fitter, healthier, functionally stronger, and more muscular body with a lower proportion of body fat than an average person would carry. However, the resultant musculature is less developed than that of a

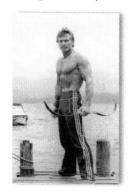

bodybuilder.

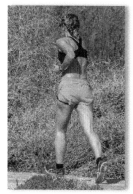

Bodybuilding is where you greatly increase the size, shape, and definition of your muscles in an aesthetically pleasing way, with many people choosing to enter contests as a result. Bodybuilders are only concerned with increased muscle size and their aesthetic shape, they're completely unconcerned about athletic ability and functional strength.

Endurance training is usually specific to athletes of all levels, both amateur and professional, who are only concerned about one thing: endurance. They're completely unconcerned about muscular size and shape, and they only require strength in relation to their chosen endurance sport.

Strength training is usually specific to athletes of all levels who are only concerned with one thing, functional 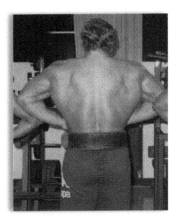 strength. As such, they usually completely ignore the aesthetic shape of their body, and the levels of body fat being carried.

All categories have one thing in common: exercise. No matter what your chosen sport or physical objective might be, it always involves some form of physical conditioning. There will always be some combination of muscular strength, size, and endurance required to participate in all sports. Naturally, this is a subject that has been thought about, debated, researched, and written about in various ways and by countless people for several millennia.

Our perspective on exercise is simple. We're only interested in the most efficient, scientific ways to achieve the results we want. To begin with we'll break down the entire process of muscle building into basic principles and descriptions.

To shape, tone, grow and strengthen your muscles, you must stimulate them enough to cause them to grow. Muscle growth is technically called hypertrophy, and it's the process which causes the cellular structure of your muscles to grow stronger and larger.

Muscle growth is your body's Adaptive Response™ from a stimulus, which is usually a workload against a resistance that is greater than what your muscles are accustomed to dealing with, and which has been applied over a certain time which is long enough to trigger the response. Working your muscles against slightly more resistance than they can normally accommodate causes them to grow in both size and strength. In growing, your muscles are compensating and adapting to meet the new demands being placed upon them.

In terms of sports, bodybuilding, and strength training, the typical form of resistance used is with weights. These are usually in the form of barbells, dumbbells, and resistance training machines. This is a very limited perspective on what constitutes a resistance. It's typically an approach adopted because people, and especially those who are new to resistance training, simply don't know any better. I'll explain more about this later.

When a muscle is exercised against a greater resistance than it can currently accommodate, tiny tissue damage occurs. This stimulates a growth in muscle size and strength to accommodate the new physical demands by overcompensating. It replaces the damaged tissue with even more tissue so that the risk of repeating the damage is going to be reduced in the future.

Within this process, something else happens which depends upon one of the following: A) the intensity of the resistance, B) the length of time which intensity is maintained, and C) whether the process has shifted from being an anaerobic process into an aerobic one.

We'll clarify what each of these means. Aerobic exercise is also known as "cardio," and this involves low to high-intensity exercise that depends primarily on the aerobic energy-generating process. Aerobic literally means: relating to, involving, or requiring free oxygen, and it refers to the use of oxygen to adequately meet the energy demands of the body during exercise. Training your muscles into the aerobic realm is better suited to people training for increased endurance, as opposed to increased strength and muscle size. Since aerobic exercise isn't especially good at shaping and building muscle mass, all body toners, body shapers, bodybuilders, and strength athletes are more focussed on anaerobic exercises. Anaerobic means without air, and that you're not using and burning air while exercising. Anaerobic exercise is achieved in periods of 60 seconds, or less, with a stimulus great enough to cause lactate to form in the muscles.

Here's the brief background about lactate, AKA: lactic acid, and how and why you'll relate to it. When you exercise, the demand for energy is high, and your body uses oxygen to break down glucose for energy. However, during extremely intense exercise, there may not be enough oxygen available to meet the demand. A substance called lactate is produced. The reason your body produced the lactate is that it can convert it into energy without using oxygen.

Lactate builds up in your bloodstream faster than you can burn it off, which then causes the burning sensation in your muscles. It's worth noting that the combination of both the micro-trauma damage, and the lactic acid formation, has been theorized as being the cause of the symptoms commonly known as Delayed Onset Muscle Soreness, or D.O.M.S.

Performing regular anaerobic exercises will help your body to more efficiently process lactic acid. In addition, there will be many other overall health-related benefits including better overall sports performance, increased metabolism, more energy, and increases in both muscle mass and bone density.

To ensure that continued progress is made in your quest to build both strength and muscle, the progressive overload method should be used. This typically means increasing the resistance being used for each exercise and reducing the rest time taken between sets of exercises. Other factors taken into practical consideration when assessing progressive improvement, might include what someone physically looks like, body fat measurements showing a reduction in the overall level, together with better blood pressure and heart readings.

Therefore, to shape, tone, and build your muscles effectively, you must exercise them in periods of 60 seconds or less, always using a resistance greater than they are used to handling, and for a long enough time. Since you now know "why" and the "how" it happens, the whole thing is simple – right?

## Bodybuilders & Strength Athletes – The Difference

One of the most frequently asked questions is, "Why do bodybuilders and strength athletes often appear so physically different?" In simple terms, they use two very different types of training regimes. These are often thought to stimulate two very different physical processes of growth to take place, but do they?

Muscle growth, AKA: hypertrophy, is currently thought to occur in either a single way or more commonly in a combination of several different ways which are:  1) through increases in the volume/size of myofibrils inside the muscles, which is commonly termed as being myofibrillar hypertrophy.  2) hyperplasia, which is when there is an increase in the number of muscle fibres. 3) sarcoplasmic growth, which is through the increase in cellular glycogen, and which results in the expansion of the fluid in the muscle.

The bottom line is that even though it's thought to exist, and there's strong evidence to suggest that it does, to date, no one has proven that pure sarcoplasmic hypertrophy exists, or not.  However, since there is a distinct difference between the functional strength of a pure bodybuilder and that of a pure strength athlete, the deeper question is: why?  More specifically, is the difference in strength between the two types of athlete primarily because of the type of resistance training each category of athlete employs or is it because the bodybuilder and the strength athlete simply focus their training towards different muscles?  Bodybuilders naturally focus a lot more on chest, shoulder and arm development, and the strength athlete focusses more on the development of the prime movers needed for heavy lifting.  This could well be one of the answers to the question.

I personally believe that the main reason why each is so typically different is due to a combination of myofibril growth, hyperplasia, together with the type of resistance training which is favoured. In addition, from the research I've seen to date, I also believe there is some validity in there being a degree of pure sarcoplasmic growth too. This may appear as though I'm sitting on the proverbial fence in this respect, and perhaps it is in some way. This is currently what I believe until I see evidence to persuade me otherwise.

We know that bodybuilders are concerned only with one thing: muscle size. Technically, bodybuilders train with a greater than normal resistance, which is typically about 60% to 80% of their one-repetition maximum. This allows them to perform sets of between 8 and 12 repetitions. They keep the rest time between each set of exercises to an absolute minimum, which then flushes, or pumps, the muscles with much more blood than normal. This is the process which is thought to cause a cellular increase in glycogen to take place. This type of muscle growth has become commonly referred to as being sarcoplasmic hypertrophy.

To clarify, glycogen is simply a type of sugar that serves as a form of energy. It's deposited in bodily tissues as a store of carbohydrates, and it's the body's main form of storage for the sugar, glucose. Glycogen is stored in two main places in the body, one being the liver, and the other being the muscles. More importantly, glycogen is the body's secondary source of long-term energy storage, with the primary energy storage source being fat. When glycogen is in the muscles, it is converted into glucose for use as energy when performing sports etc., and glycogen stored in the liver is converted into glucose for use as energy throughout the body, and in the central nervous system.

The glycogen in the muscle cells keeps them both hydrated (pumped) and expanded, with between three and four parts of water. This is perfect for bodybuilders because their entire focus of training is to create extremely large muscles 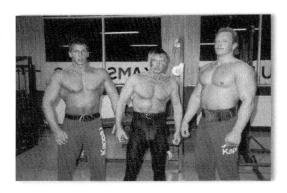 that are aesthetically pleasing in terms of size, shape, balance, and muscular definition. Any gains in functional muscle strength for bodybuilders is merely a by-product of the bodybuilding process. It's certainly not the end-focus. Bodybuilders don't typically focus their training solely on the prime mover muscles which the strength athletes do, because other muscles must be developed to achieve an overall balanced appearance. This is almost certainly the main reason why bodybuilders often tend to be functionally weaker than their massively muscular physical appearance suggests. Even a bodybuilder who is comparatively weaker than a pure strength athlete is still enormously strong when compared to someone who doesn't exercise at all.

Conversely, strength training isn't focussed in any way whatsoever on muscle size or shape. Instead, it's entirely focussed on increases in functional strength. Strength athletes typically exercise with greater resistances than bodybuilders. They use between 80% and 90% of their one-repetition maximum, which allows sets of between only 1 and 6 repetitions per exercise to be performed.

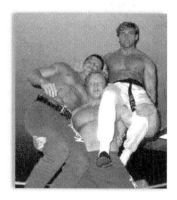

The rest time between the sets of exercises is also much longer than for bodybuilders and can last several minutes.

Exercising this way will stimulate deep tissue growth, with both myofibril hypertrophy and hyperplasia taking place. Both forms of hypertrophy result in an increase in functional strength, and the approach is typical of professional strength athletes, powerlifters, and Olympic weight-lifters.

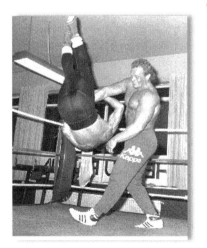

As we know, when a muscle is exercised in this way, against a near-maximum resistance compared to what it can currently handle, micro-trauma occurs in the muscle tissue. Technically, this is damage being

190

caused to the tiny muscle fibres, or sarcomeres. The sarcomeres must adapt to the new demands being placed upon them by increasing their size. Inside each of the tiny sarcomeres, a special interaction takes place. This interaction is between the myosin molecules and a protein cross-bridge called actin. This interaction only takes place when sufficient micro-trauma, or damage, has occurred.

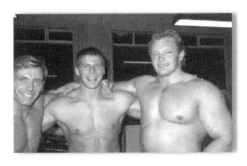

With sufficient micro-trauma, combined with enough recovery time and sufficient nutrition, the myosin and actin in the damaged areas attract new growth elements to help them accommodate the increased demands being placed upon them. The result is that they grow thicker and with stronger filaments than before, causing the sarcomeres to expand in size as the amount of myosin and actin increases. Increasing the size, density, and quantity of the muscle fibres will naturally produce a significant increase in overall strength.

Pure bodybuilders and pure strength athletes often differ so much in size and shape. They've simply focussed more of their training efforts on stimulating one aspect of muscle growth.

Naturally, none of the processes of hypertrophy happens in pure isolation. They always occur in a combination of ways, with the chosen type of training

191

always leaning towards one type of muscle growth. This is a cross-over effect, and it's one that produces a balance of muscle growth and increases in functional muscle strength. The choice of that balance is entirely up to the individual concerned, and which method of exercise they've been biased towards during their training.

There are people who believe that isometric exercise will make you stronger, however, they also believe that it won't produce an increase in muscle size. Naturally, this is complete nonsense. Certain types of exercise may produce a greater, or a lesser degree, of increased muscle size, but there will always be an 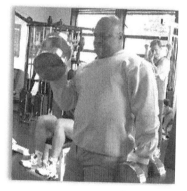 increase. People who suggest otherwise should stop and think for a moment about the physics of material science.

Taking a steel cable as an example. There is always going to be a limit to the lifting capacity of any specific diameter of steel cable. Increase the diameter of the cable, and you can lift more weight with it. The same is true of muscle. Once a critical mass point has been reached, the human body naturally increases the size and density of the muscle to accommodate the increased demands being placed upon it. Isometric exercise is no different to any other kind of resistance training. If a muscle is sufficiently stimulated, then it will grow larger, and stronger as a result. Isometric exercise is simply a method of very efficiently producing the required stimulus.

### Endurance Athletes

There's one other type of sportsperson: the endurance athlete.
Since the goals of endurance athletes are very different to both pure strength athletes, and pure bodybuilders, they use a very different 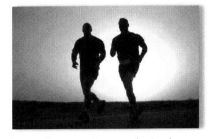 approach to achieve the balanced musculature their chosen sports require. In resistance training, endurance athletes would typically use between 40% and 60% of their one repetition maximum resistance. They would perform a minimum of 12 repetitions per exercise, for several sets of each exercise, and with minimum rest time between each set. This gives them the balance of muscle strength, and muscular endurance they need. At the same time, it minimises the possibility of increases in muscle size because significant muscle growth would almost always be an impediment in their chosen sports.

### Strength, Stamina, Endurance, and Resilience

It is important to understand the difference between strength, stamina and endurance because once understood, you'll then be able to devise the most suitable workout routines according to your body type.

Muscular strength is possibly best understood as being a muscle's capacity to exert force against resistance, or weight. This is comparatively easy to measure because your ability to lift a given amount of weight for a single repetition is a good measure of your strength.

Stamina is the length of time at which a muscle, or group of muscles, can perform at or near your maximum capacity. For example, the number of squats you can perform with a given weight which is 90% of your maximum would be a measure of your stamina or the distance which you can carry a similarly heavy object such as an anvil.

Endurance is all about time, and your ability to perform a certain muscular action for a prolonged period regardless of the capacity at which you're working.

Resilience is all about your ability to recover from whatever stresses and demands are placed upon your muscles. However, resilience is mostly all about your state of mind, your mental toughness and ability to endure, perform and deliver under pressure, and to recover quickly emotionally.

The muscular composition of your body will always determine how well you will perform at certain sports. The amount of slow twitch muscle fibres you possess will determine how well you perform at endurance related events, and both type A and type B fast twitch muscle fibres are all about explosive power and your ability to maintain it.

If you possess mostly slow twitch fibres, then you're naturally better suited to endurance sports. Alternatively, if you possess mostly fast twitch muscle fibres, then you're a natural weightlifter. It's important to note, that no matter what your natural predisposition might be in this respect, with the correct training regimen, it is still possible to significantly increase your abilities in your naturally weaker opposing areas of speciality.

### Workout Intensity

When you exercise, the intensity which is delivered into the exercise being performed is a vital factor which should always be considered, no matter what your objectives might be. How hard is hard? How intense is intense? These are both very subjective things. Taking two people of equal fitness, something that is intense and tough to one person might be considered comparatively easy to another. The only factor differentiating between the two is usually going to be mental toughness and determination.

In addition to this, your brain has a built-in mechanism which helps to protect the body and prevent it from performing physical activity to such a level that could cause serious damage or even death to be the result. This is the mechanism that makes your brain tell you to stop exercising when it begins to get tough, and the feeling only increases as you continue to push yourself, even though you're physically capable of doing much, much more.

The brain of people who exercise regularly, and especially to a high level of intensity, will somehow naturally adjust this safety margin marker over time. This means that their

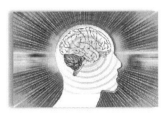 brain doesn't tell them to stop an exercise until the level of intensity being reached is much higher than it would be for a beginner. When it comes to exercise, how is it possible to impart various levels of recommended intensity, especially when to some degree these are always going to be subjective to the individual?

Scientists think they have found a way to solve this problem. It's called Transcranial Magnetic Stimulation, or TMS for short. Transcranial Magnetic Stimulation is a non-invasive method that uses electromagnetic coils placed against the scalp to measure and assess the levels of stress and fatigue caused by resistance training and other forms of exercise. TMS can accurately assess the level of fatigue in the brain's motor cortex, and when professional athletes are monitored, it's a way coaches can determine just how intense the workout load really is, compared to what an athlete is capable of. It's also a good way to determine when to reduce an athlete's load, and/or training frequency, to prevent overtraining before it becomes a serious problem.

So, what does this mean when it comes to determining how to accurately communicate levels of

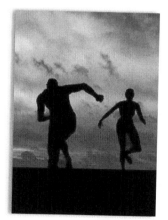

exercise intensity, especially when there's no professional coach or elaborate and expensive equipment at hand? The most obvious thing about this research is that it means almost everyone will stop exercising LONG before they're in any danger of becoming seriously fatigued. In other words, most people will *think* themselves into achieving much less intensity than they're capable of if they were just a little more mentally resilient. This doesn't mean that people should suddenly begin pushing themselves way beyond their physical limits, which would be nothing short of stupid. What it does mean though, is that most people who enjoy a higher than average mental resilience and determination, as well as being in physically good condition, can push themselves much harder than they might think.

Naturally, if anyone ever feels "genuine" strain or fatigue to the point of becoming injured, then they should stop exercising immediately. It also further strengthens the reasons why EVERYONE should always seek medical approval from their physician before undertaking any form of exercise or following any kind of new diet plan.

## *Training Hard for Hours – The Myth*

We're amazed by how many supposedly intelligent people still try to convince us that they spend an hour, or more, in a gym, and during that entire time they're training at the highest intensity possible. That's complete and utter rubbish. There's just no other way to say it. If you're one of these people who believes this, then shame on you, because the science is simple and extremely clear in this respect. Here's the bad news, you can't change the laws of physics or biology to substantiate your ridiculous rhetoric.

If you really do train as hard as humanly possible, with near 100% maximum intensity, which involves super-strict form, training to complete failure, negatives reps, and perhaps even performing assisted repetitions (not just assisted because you're lazy and lack willpower), then you simply can't train for a long period of time. It's physiologically impossible unless you're an alien from the planet which exists only in movies and comic books, and you wear the letter 'S' on a dodgy looking "onesie leotard," and with your underwear "suspiciously" on the outside of your costume. I may be joking a little here, however, I'm completely serious in what I say about training hard.

The physics are simple. The intensity of your workout is directly proportional to the length of time that you're physically able to perform your workout. The harder and more intensely you exercise, then the shorter time that you'll be physically able to perform the exercise, it's just basic physics and biology.

Think about a car as an analogy. If you rev the engine hard and work it to the absolute maximum, then it will wear much more quickly than it would do by simply revving it more gently. Just as with almost everything in life, the harder that you work it, or use it, then the shorter the length of time that it lasts. If you've been "one of those embarrassing people" who've tried to "sell" others on the idea that you're somehow different and can work at maximum intensity for hours on end, then stop right now. Everyone knows that you're talking complete rubbish, and it's embarrassing for your family and friends who are forced to listen to you. They're just being nice to you when they "pretend" to listen intently to your drivel, while at the same time trying not to laugh at you. You may as well try to convince people that "Pigs might fly if they only had wings," which is an old British response to people talking complete rubbish.

## Ultra-High Intensity Training – Ultra-Short Bursts

The benefits of short, highly intense exercise sessions are becoming increasingly reported in credible newsfeeds across the world, and two such reports were recently published by the British National Health Service.

One report was about the results of scientific experiments conducted by Dr Jonathan Little et al, from McMaster University in Canada, and it was published in the Journal of Physiology. This is the same university where the eminent sports physiologist, Professor Martin Gibala and his team performed their ground-breaking research into the benefits of high-intensity exercise. In the report, it concluded that one of the best ways to keep fit was to do less exercise, rather than more. It found that regular, short, and highly intense workout sessions were more than enough to keep most people fit and healthy. The research completely overturned the long-standing theory that it takes hours of exercise dedication to stay in shape.

Other similar studies were performed by researchers from the K.G. Jebsen Centre for Exercise in Medicine in Norway, and at other research centres in Norway, Canada, and the USA. The research found that as little as 12 minutes of comparatively intense exercise a week, was all that was needed to improve a person's overall health, fitness, and strength. They also found that short, intense exercise sessions were very effective in increasing a person's Base Metabolic Rate and aiding in overall weight loss.

Perhaps the most impactful research was carried out by Professor Jamie Timmons of Nottingham University in England, who conducted a four-year detailed study with over 1000 test subjects. The conclusions which Professor Timmons and his team reached were remarkable.

Unsurprisingly, they found that the key to gaining the greatest benefits from exercise was in extremely short high-intensity sessions, and not in lengthy, prolonged workouts. Their research also concluded that as little as 3 minutes per week of extremely high-intensity exercise, performed in only very short bursts, is all that's needed to significantly boost a person's Base Metabolic Rate (BMR), dramatically improve cardiovascular efficiency, and improve their overall health. HIIT, or High-Intensity Interval Training was just one of the ways which were investigated, and it was proven to be of enormous benefit in terms of health and fitness.

The benefits of HIIT were first discovered by Professor Martin Gibala and his team at McMaster University, in Canada. They began what we now call "the exercise revolution" when they found that HIIT delivered the same physical benefits as traditional endurance training, but in a considerably shorter time, and with less exercise. Later, Professor Gibala and his team found that less extreme forms of HIIT worked just as well for people who weren't already good athletes, who were older, and who were overweight and unfit. However, even in the less intense form of HIIT, the workout was still beyond the general comfort zone of most people, but it was still far less than a serious athlete's maximum capacity.

Therefore, by default, the ISOfitness™ system is a fusion of two extremely well researched, and scientific proven exercise systems. One is the isometric exercise system, in which exercises are most effective when they're performed in high-intensity bursts of between 7 and 10 seconds. The seconds is the proven superior health, fitness, and wellness benefits of very short bursts of extremely high-intensity exercise, as researched and proven by Professor Timmons, Professor Gibala, and others. The ISOfitness™ exercise system is all about what we call **U**ltra-**H**igh **I**ntensity **T**raining - **U**ltra-**S**hort **B**urst™ exercise sessions, AKA: UHIT-USB™.

## *Why is UHIT-USB™ so Effective?*

How does it all work? Firstly, traditional HIIT engages much more muscle tissue than traditional aerobic exercise, and when you engage upper body muscles as well as lower body muscles in bursts of high-intensity exercise, as much as 80% of the body's overall muscle cells are engaged. This is massive, especially when compared to more traditional aerobic exercises such as jogging or cycling, which only engages somewhere between 20% and 40% of the body's overall muscle cells at best.

Short bursts of high-intensity exercise also do something else, they're exactly what's needed to break down the body's stored reserves of glucose in the muscles, which is called glycogen. When these reserves of glycogen are rapidly depleted due to the high-intensity bursts of exercise, it creates room for the glucose in your blood to replace it and be stored instead. In short, it removes some of the sugar circulating in your bloodstream, which in turn has both overall health and weight loss benefits.

Exercises in the ISOfitness™ system are all about ultra-high intensity training performed in ultra-short bursts. They're the natural evolution of the two proven scientific methods. When combined, these two methods produce even better results than they did as individual and separate concepts. All exercises in the ISOfitness™ system are performed in a maximum of 10 seconds, which is exactly the time that Professor Timmons and his team found to be optimal for each burst of extremely high-intensity exercise. That's the exact same amount of time that is in direct accordance with the masses of the proven science behind Isometric contraction exercise. We explain the science behind this in much greater detail in a later section.

Another factor which can also be taken into consideration, especially for more advanced athletes, is rest time. According to the highly acclaimed and pioneering sports scientist, Arthur Jones, the man who invented the famous Nautilus system, muscle recovery has a half-life which occurs every 3 seconds after an exercise has been stopped. This means that advanced sports enthusiasts, bodybuilders, and even professional athletes, can factor-in the "exercise half-life" concept, to produce the most effective exercise regimen targeted to their needs. If muscle recovery has a half-life which occurs every 3 seconds, then after only 9 seconds, you're technically ready to perform your next exercise or set of exercises.

## *In Practical Terms*

We've now explored in an overview format, the concepts surrounding rest time, exercise half-life, "how hard is hard," workout intensity, and that there are very specific, and very different training methods that can be employed to achieve specific goals. We've also established that each of the different methods will have an equally different effect on overall muscle size, shape, endurance, and functional ability. In addition to this, we've also now established that there are specific differences between how pure bodybuilders, strength athletes, and endurance athletes will train.

Therefore, what does all this mean in practical terms to someone who wishes to train for one of the categories listed above, or for a combination of categories? Where, and how, do people usually start their training? Unsurprisingly, most people will join a gym or fitness club, depending upon the local vernacular. In the better clubs, there will usually be some sort of induction course, which will orientate and familiarise the new member to the basics of resistance training.

In the "not-so-good" clubs, people are usually expected to either already know what to do, or they are forced to watch the other gym members and copy them in some way. The induction courses are usually more about the gym covering their back legally, to "appear" to have taught new members what to do, and in doing so, keeping their insurance company happy.

It's simply impossible to teach an absolute beginner how to work-out properly during the short time-span of even the world's best gym induction course. Unless the new member already knows about proper exercise methods, they must continually ask what to do. This isn't always made easy, because the people who work in the gyms would much prefer their new clients to book private coaching sessions with them, rather than give advice for free. It's common to see people in gyms performing a variety of weird and wonderful exercises, usually in appalling style.

Perhaps the funniest thing about it all, is that all the machines in gyms almost always have clearly written

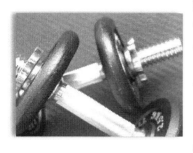

instruction cards attached to the frames, complete with descriptive pictures and narratives. Therefore, if followed, even a complete beginner won't find it too hard to navigate through and to get a reasonable workout. Despite these clearly written instructions and pictures, many people who become gym members seem to suffer from the "Dunning-Kruger Effect" I mentioned earlier, of being too stupid to realise that they're stupid. The result is that if there's a completely wrong way to perform an exercise, they'll find it, and do it. However, by some miracle, even those who fall into the category described above, often still manage to achieve some reasonable results DESPITE what they do. It makes you wonder just how much more they'd achieve if they only used just a fraction more common sense.

If you decide to join a gym and hire a good coach, then you'll usually achieve some good results. Your coach will devise a routine which would vary the exercises, combinations of resistance used, number repetitions performed, and the number of sets. This would combine to help ensure that your workout routine doesn't become predictable and stale. You'll make steady progress toward your objective. To summarise, the traditional approaches to resistance training requires that you always have the following:

▲ A gym membership of some sort, which can be expensive. You may be lucky enough to have enough space, and money, to equip a professional standard home gym. However, this is rare.

▲ Professional coaching, proper instruction about exercise, meal plans, and a good workout strategy.

▲ Enough of the right resistance equipment. All gyms vary in the quality, quantity, and standard of equipment. This is usually in the form of barbells, dumbbells, and weight discs. Various machines are also used, some of which are disc loaded, while others have selector weight stacks.

▲ Time. You'll need time to spend in the gym, travelling there, and home again, often in busy traffic in either one or both parts of your journey.

Whichever way you look at it, getting into shape requires that you'll commit a large portion of your free time, and a considerable sum of money. Change doesn't always come for free. If you're clever about it, then you really don't need to spend fortunes on achieving your goals, nor do you need to use up all your free time.

To achieve excellent results in a non-traditional way, it requires that you're able to think laterally, you're non-judgemental, and that you have an open mind. You also must be prepared to try an exercise system which some people don't give much of a thought to anymore, typically because it's not considered to be "sexy," or more usually because they just don't understand them. However, it's an exercise system that has been scientifically proven to deliver outstanding results, faster than any of the other methods.

## Chapter 6: The Science of Exercise

There are three basic types of resistance training. One type is isometric. These are exercises performed without involving any measurable movement of the limb that is being exercised. The second type is isotonic exercise, which is all about movement. The third is isokinetic, which is about movement, however, with certain modifications to standard isotonic exercise applying to speed, velocity and force. Isokinetic exercises are not as common as traditional isotonic exercises.

An exercise is isotonic when the tension remains the same, whilst the length of the muscle changes, such as when lifting and lowering a weight. There are two types of isotonic contractions: concentric (lifting) and eccentric (lowering). In a concentric contraction, the muscle tension rises to meet the resistance, then remains the same as the muscle shortens. In the eccentric, the muscle lengthens due to the resistance being greater than the force the muscle is producing.

Isokinetic and isotonic contractions appear to be the same, however, they are technically very different. During exercise, an isotonic contraction will keep force at a constant, while velocity changes. An isokinetic contraction will keep velocity at a constant, while the force changes.

An exercise is isometric when a muscle or a group of muscles are contracted to exert a force against an immovable object. The muscles will then remain fixed in that specific position for the entire duration of the exercise, and the associated joint doesn't move either.

### Isotonic Exercise Elaborated

The traditional isotonic exercises are more commonly known as either weight training or bodyweight-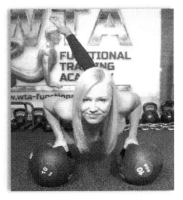only resistance-based exercises. In weight training, it's obvious that it's the weights in the form of barbells, dumbbells, and machines, which provide the resistance needed to exercise the muscles. In bodyweight-only exercises, it's also equally obvious that a person's own bodyweight and limb-leverage provides the resistance needed to exercise the muscles.

As a footnote, resistance machines have one huge drawback, together with one reasonable advantage when compared to the use of both weights and bodyweight-only exercises. This is because when you use a machine, your body is typically secured and stabilised in either a seat or on a bench. This means that your body isn't using many of the core supporting muscles to lift the weights.

Instead, the focus is entirely on strengthening the comparatively small, isolated muscle groups that the machine is targeting. The result is that your overall functional body strength is going to be impaired, and because your core musculature isn't being strengthened, you will also be more susceptible to an increased risk of injury. The main advantage that resistance machines provide is that they usually have the added benefit of

207

incorporating built-in off-set cams. These cams provide a more evenly balanced resistance curve throughout the exercise movement.

This is because it provides extra resistance to your muscles during the comparatively easier part of the exercise. Since every limb of the body is just like a machine, and the rules of basic mechanical leverage also govern the limbs of the human body. This means that at certain angles, every limb finds it easier to lift a weight than it does at other angles. This is known as either mechanical advantage or mechanical disadvantage.

In basic weight training using barbells and dumbbells, the force you exert is kept constant against the chosen resistance, and it's only the velocity which changes through a specific range of motion during the exercise.

When a full-range repetition of any traditional resistance exercise is performed, such as the barbell curl, biomechanical changes as well as speed and velocity all

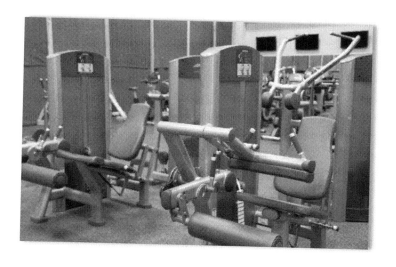

come into play as factors which can affect the absolute engagement of the muscle being exercised.

Taking the barbell curl as an example, the exercise is performed as follows. Standing upright and holding a barbell with both hands in a hanging position in front of you, the barbell is lifted by bending the arms upwards, while ensuring that the elbows don't move forward, or away from the side of the body. This movement is intended to isolate and work the

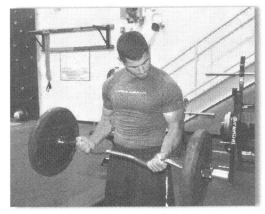

biceps muscles. In the upper position, which is the end of the first part of the movement, the bar is roughly at shoulder height. In that position, there is a slight pause before the bar is then returned slowly, and under control, to the starting position so that the exercise can either be repeated or stopped.

In traditional resistance training, most people and even supposedly reputable coaches, completely fail to realise that it's the lowering, AKA: the negative, eccentric part of the movement, which is much more beneficial to muscle growth than the concentric, AKA: the lifting part. During the eccentric part of any resistance training exercise, many beneficial things happen. This includes the stimulation and engagement of more muscle fibres, and especially fast-twitch fibres, increases in neural pathway stimulation, and a greater micro-trauma to the sarcomeres. Perhaps there's nothing very surprising in any of that. Performing a movement which is resisted by a weight will eventually result in developing muscles which are larger, stronger, more toned, and ultimately more aesthetically pleasing in size and shape than they were before. Focussing on performing a slower eccentric motion, produces stronger and bigger muscles, than if you focus on the concentric part of the exercise. This is because the new chemical bonds produced because of the eccentric motion are very strong, which directly result in longer lasting muscle and strength gains.

## Super-Slow Training

Super Slow is a form of strength training which was made popular by Ken Hutchins who worked at Nautilus. However, it is based on an original concept by Dr Vincent Bocchicchio. He proposed that a single repetition of resistance training should take 10 seconds for the lifting phase, which is the concentric contraction where the muscles shorten, and then after a slight pause to prevent momentum being generated, taking another 10 seconds for the lowering, or eccentric phase, where the muscles lengthen.

The super-slow concept incorporates extremely slow repetition speeds when compared to traditional resistance training protocols. In super-slow training, the emphasis is on minimizing momentum through minimal acceleration which improves muscular loading. Most research suggests that super-slow training yields better results in terms of strength gains and muscle growth than traditional resistance training methods.

The heart of the super-slow concept is based on the amount of tension a muscle develops. This is directly affected by the speed at which the muscle lengthens during the eccentric or lowering phase or shortens during the concentric or lifting phase of an exercise.

The more tension that is generated, the more muscle fibres that are recruited. More importantly, the slower the myosin and actin filaments within the muscle fibres slide past each other, the more links that are formed between the filaments. Therefore, using super-slow exercise speeds a maximum amount of tension is generated and a higher number of filament links are formed. In short, super-slow training activates more muscle fibres at an increased rate to maintain the force necessary to move the resistance provided. This is why it is a very efficient way to increase both strength and muscle size.

A typical super-slow workout would consist of one set of each exercise which is performed to the point of complete muscle fatigue/failure. Therefore, a 10-repetition exercise in such a routine would take between 200 and 250 seconds to perform in practice, with the overall workouts session taking no longer than 30 minutes to complete. Since this is a high-intensity system, it requires greater rest time between workout sessions. Therefore, a workout frequency of twice each week is typically recommended.

One of the great advantages of super-slow training is in injury prevention. This is because in traditional resistance training, to make it more challenging more force is required through and increased resistance/weight being used.  Therefore, the traditional method naturally increases the risk of injury.  However, with super-slow training, you can make the exercise more challenging and engage more muscle fibres without increasing the force/weight.

A by-product of super-slow training is that it provides excellent cardiovascular benefits.  This is because the heart is an involuntary muscle, therefore, it will always pump harder when there is more blood which needs pumping.  Several studies have shown that super-slow training returns more blood to the heart than traditional aerobic training methods.

## Callisthenics

Just like weight training, callisthenics are a form of isotonic training.  There are several methods of exercise that are a viable satisfactory alternative to a traditional gym-based exercise routine.  The first that comes to mind is a basic freehand callisthenic routine.  A callisthenic routine simply means bodyweight-only exercises of various kinds, such as push-ups, pull-ups, squats, lunges, trunk curls, and dips etc.  The word "callisthenics" is derived from a combination of the ancient Greek words "kalos," which means "perfect," and "sthenos," meaning "strength."

These exercises are excellent at building and maintaining levels of high levels of fitness, balance, endurance, and a considerable degree of strength.  There are certain callisthenic exercises which can develop great strength, such as the ones used by gymnasts.  These are primarily pull-ups, dips, and handstand dips.

During the gymnastic-style exercises, the gymnast performing them would adjust the speed, velocity, and the angles that the exercise is typically performed at, which usually significantly increases the level of difficulty. These exercises almost always include a portion of isometric, or static, exercise-hold as well.

There is a serious drawback to advanced callisthenics being a complete substitute for a gym-based strength workout. This is that for most people without excellent gymnastic skills, once you've become accustomed to handling your own body weight when performing the various exercises, then you need to use techniques to place you at a biomechanical disadvantage to gain increased resistance.

In addition, you need a certain degree of equipment available, and/or similarly improvised facilities to allow a gymnastic-style workout routine to be performed. At the very least, you'll need equipment or facilities to perform pull-ups and dips. If you don't have these, then unless you find another way of applying more resistance through biomechanical disadvantage during each exercise, then you're primarily only performing a basic fitness/resilience/endurance routine. You're almost certainly not performing a resistance routine that is focussed on growing strength and muscle.

The other major drawback is that you need a certain degree of space to perform an effective gymnastic-style callisthenics workout routine. Therefore, you can't really perform any exercise easily, and relatively unobtrusively in a public or semi-public place.

## *Isokinetic Training*

Isokinetic is a type of calisthenic exercise, or exercise involving movement, that takes place at a constant speed no matter how much effort is exerted. The word, "isokinetic" comes from a combination of ancient Greek and Latin. The word "Isos" means: same/equal, and the word "kinesis" means motion or movement.

One of the main advantages of isokinetic exercise is that the muscles being exercised gain strength evenly throughout the full range of movement of the limb being exercised. Also, a great deal of research suggests that isokinetic training is one of the most efficient ways to increase strength and build muscle. This could also be due, at least in part, to the slower exercise speeds being used while generating maximum tension/force for each repetition of an exercise.

One of the typical disadvantages of isokinetic training is that it typically requires special exercise equipment that is very expensive. This is because the equipment has to sense when a movement is increasing in speed so that it then automatically increases the resistance in order to slow it down and maintain the desired constant speed for the exercise.

To a certain degree, the development and implementation of the popular off-set elliptical cams in most modern exercise machines is an inexpensive albeit much less efficient, way of addressing this issue. It's also worth remembering that most isokinetic exercises can be performed very effectively with an Iso-Bow®.

### *Isometric Exercise Elaborated*

Isometric exercise is very different to traditional isotonic resistance training because isometric exercises do not involve any movement. Instead, an exercise is isometric when a muscle, or a group of muscles, are contracted to exert a force against an immovable object. The muscles being exercised then remain fixed in a specific position for the entire duration of the exercise, and the associated joint doesn't move either. If required, an isometric contraction exercise can then be repeated at various positions throughout each limb's entire range of motion.

If you want to be hyper-technical, there is always going to be some very slight movement involved in any isometric exercise. This is because when a muscle is contracted against an immovable object there will always be some micro-movement involving the contraction of the muscles, and a slight bending of the bones etc. That's only something the "nit-pickers" would point out, and that's as far is it goes in respect of any movement being involved.

The term "isometric" has Greek origins, and it's derived from combining two words, one of which is "isos," which means: "equal," and the other being "metria," meaning: measuring. It's also part of the etymological root of the word "metre" in the metric system of measurement. In English, the word "isometric" means: "equal distance," or "equal measurement." In addition to this, the term "static," or "statics" have often been used throughout history to describe what we now call the Isometric system of exercise. The word "static" comes to the English language through Latin "staticus," from the Greek word "statikos" which means: "causing to stand." In language terms from an exercise perspective, the term "static" or "statics" has the same meaning as "isometric."

Between 1953 and 1958, one of the most extensive research studies ever undertaken was performed at the world-famous Max Plank Institute in Dortmund, Germany. These are now considered by many to be the original "gold standard" of all exercise studies. It's perhaps best remembered and known about, because of the resultant ground-breaking book: "The Physiology of Strength," by Dr Theodor Hettinger - Research Fellow at the Max Plank Institute.

During that 5-year research period, over 5,500 experiments were performed on volunteers from all walks of life, and at every level of strength and fitness. This broad spectrum of test subjects included serious strength athletes, and middle-aged, generally unfit people. The conclusion of these studies proved beyond doubt, the overall superiority of isometric exercise.

The Max Plank research study also revealed something perhaps even more remarkable. This was that after performing only one single training stimulus per day, the muscle being exercised was no longer responsive to further gains. The scientific data about this can be referenced on pages 28 to 31 of Dr Theodor Hettinger's book "The Physiology of Strength."

In other words, performing only one single isometric contraction exercise, lasting for 7 seconds, was the all the exercise that was needed to produce the maximum strength gains possible for each muscle group exercised. The research also showed that it didn't matter how many additional isometric exercise holds were performed, the initial, single 7-second exercise was all that was needed.

In addition, there were remarkable gains in strength documented. For example, a single, daily 7-second isometric exercise, when performed at absolute maximum intensity, could produce a staggering 14% increase in strength per day. The scientific data about this can be referenced on page 30 of Dr Theodor Hettinger's book "The Physiology of Strength." Another group studied by Dr Hettinger and Dr Muller who trained at close to 100% of their maximum capacity once each day, achieved an astonishing increase in muscle size and strength of over 12%. Both sets of test results are exceptional, even by the highest of professional standards.

Naturally, both practical, and experimental results will always vary slightly according to the individuals concerned, recovery methods, rest time, and nutrition. As discussed in the section about workout intensity, without an array of testing equipment and physiologists on hand, the question of exactly what constitutes "maximum" is always going to be somewhat subjective.

We should consider this to be an effort producing intensity at such a level that completely exhausts the individual performing the exercise. There's no escaping it, exerting 100% maximum effort in an isometric contraction lasting between 6 and 7 seconds is extremely exhausting, and it's something that is only possible to be performed safely by advanced athletes and professional sports people.

217

The scientific research studies by Dr Hettinger and Dr Muller concluded something far more practical and useful for the average person. Their studies revealed that by performing only one daily isometric exercise for a period of between 6 and 7 seconds, and at only 2/3$^{rd}$'s of an individual's maximum effort, it had the ability to increase strength by an average of up to 5% per week. By any standards, strength gains of 5% in exchange for the expenditure of only 60%, or around 2/3$^{rd}$'s of an individual's maximum capacity, is an excellent result.

This is especially impressive when one also considers that there will be an accompanying increase in muscle size, improvements in overall body shape, and functional strength. More importantly, these results are far superior to the results gained through traditional weight training. They are also results that are easily attainable, even for a complete beginner to achieve.

Since then, scientists and sports physiologists became increasingly interested in the remarkable results it was possible to achieve through Isometric exercise. Many other subsequent studies were then performed by reputable scientists at leading universities, and they all reported similar results. These include Gardner 1963, Bender 1963, Raitsin 1974, Lindh 1979, Thérpaut Mathieu 1988, Kitai 2001, and Kanehisa 2002.

Some of the studies listed above documented even greater percentage increases in strength compared to those found in the original experiments conducted by Dr Hettinger and Dr Muller. The new research revealed that it was possible to achieve improvements in muscle size, and strength, in a range of between 14% and a staggering 40%.

In 2001, Nicolas Babault PhD of the University of Burgundy, Dijon, France, led a team of scientists to research and examine how many muscle fibres were activated, and how long they remained active for, during both traditional weight training and in isometric training.

(*The scientific research paper is published: Nicolas Babault, Michel Pousson, Yves Ballay, and Jacques Van Hoecke - Groupe Analyse du Mouvement, Unite´ de Formation et de Recherche Sciences et Techniques des Activite´s Physiques et Sportives, Universite´ de Bourgogne, BP 27877, 21078 Dijon Cedex, France.*)

The research study revealed that levels of muscle activation during repetitions of maximal weight training were between 89.7%, during the concentric contraction, or the lifting a weight, and 88.3% during the eccentric contraction, or the lowering of a weight.  For practical purposes, about 89% overall.

The scientific measurement also showed that during the lifting, AKA: concentric, part of the exercise, the maximum intramuscular tension only lasted for between 0.25 and 0.5 seconds.  For practical purposes, about 1/3rd of a second overall.  This is because traditional isotonic resistance exercises involve movement, so they also have velocity and acceleration aspects to consider.  Furthermore, "force" is only produced for split seconds to produce a maximal contraction of the muscle fibres.

The research revealed that during isometric exercise, the levels of muscle activation were higher than it is in traditional isotonic resistance exercise. In fact, muscle fibre activation was as high as 95.2%, and it also lasted far longer than it did in weight training.

Maximal isometric contraction recruits nearly all the muscle motor units, and for a greater length of time than in traditional resistance exercises. Since the optimum time to perform an isometric contraction is 7 seconds, then the muscle activation also lasted for that time, which is a huge increase over the $1/3^{rd}$ of second muscular activation achieved during a single repetition of traditional weight training.

I'll use a regular dumbbell curl exercise as my example. The objective is to engage as many muscle fibres possible with each repetition, to create a maximum muscular contraction when you perform the exercise.

The level of muscle activation during this, and in any other weight training exercise, will for practical terms be 89% overall, and maximum muscular contraction will only last for approximately $1/3^{rd}$ of a second per repetition. This means that after performing 10 near-perfect high-intensity repetitions of the curl, it will still only produce around 89% maximum muscular engagement for a total only 3.3 seconds.

In contrast, I'll use an equivalent isometric biceps curl exercise, and take the 10 seconds as the typical isometric contraction exercise time. This is because it's the exercise time most often used, and the most often suggested by many expert isometric coaches to compensate for exercise engagement variables etc.

During this equivalent isometric exercise, the levels of muscle fibre activation will be as high as a massive 95.2%, and it also lasts for the full 10 seconds of the isometric exercise time. This means that a single, 10-second isometric exercise is equal to as many as 30 repetitions of near-perfect high-intensity regular weight training.

Another significant experiment was conducted by Dr Hiroaki Kanehisa et al (2002) in the Department of Life Science (Sports Sciences) at University of Tokyo, Japan, about the effects of Isometric Training Programs on Muscle Size and Strength.

Over a 10-week course of research, and with test subjects training only 3 times per week, it showed there were significant muscle volume and strength gains in two test groups. One test group performed isometric contractions at 100% of their individual maximum capacity, and the other test group trained at only 60% of their individual maximum capacity.

Perhaps unsurprisingly, the results of Dr. Kanehisa's research clearly showed that the group performing isometric contractions at 100% of their individual maximum capacity had achieved a 12.4% increase in both muscle strength and size, as opposed to a still very respectable 5.3% increase in muscle strength and size for the 60% intensity group.

More importantly, the results of Dr Kanehisa's studies clearly supported and substantiated the original conclusions of the extensive studies performed by Dr Hettinger and Dr Muller in their ground-breaking research many years earlier.

It should also be noted that many other studies have recorded a direct link to the ability to apply different levels of intensity, the length of time which an isometric

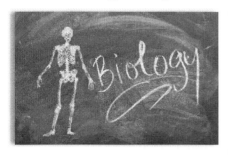

exercise can and should be held at each of those levels.  For example, if 2/3$^{rd}$'s, or approximately between 60 and 70% intensity is applied, then the time for the exercise will be 7 seconds.  There is a directly proportionate link between time, intensity, and the ability to apply that intensity.

This means that the greater the intensity applied, the less time the exercise can be performed for, and in indeed needs to be performed, to get maximum results. Therefore, at 80 to 90% of maximum intensity, some research has suggested that the exercise lasts for around 5 seconds, and at a genuine 100%, an exercise should be held for between 2 and 3 seconds.

The fact is that isometric exercises are much more scientific in their application, and approach.  They're also much more efficient than traditional resistance training, and they engage many more muscle fibres over a much longer length of time.

Since the optimum time to perform an isometric hold is 7 seconds, then this is 6.7 seconds more than a regular single repetition of traditional resistance training, which at best only engages the muscle fibres for about 1/3$^{rd}$

of a second.  During the 7 second exercise period, the intensity and focus generated stimulated and engaged almost all the type 2 fibres in the muscle to the point of failure.  These are the type of fibres that must be targeted in order to grow stronger and bigger muscles.

## *Strength at Only One Angle?*

A common myth is that isometric contraction exercises only increases muscle strength at the specific angle at which the muscle and joint are exercised.  When talking about building strength in a broader range, rather than at a more specific point, one of the first things that should also be remembered is that during regular isotonic weight training, a constant-curve range of strength gain isn't achieved anyway.

Furthermore, this issue isn't as easily resolved using traditional isotonic resistance equipment as it is by performing isometric contraction exercises.   The data clearly shows that in respect of isometric exercise, it's only partially true that there's only an increase in strength at the angle the contraction is engaged.

The scientific study performed by scientists Kitai and Sale called: "Specificity of Joint Angle in Isometric Training," concluded that strength gains were the greatest at the specific angle the training was performed.  It also concluded that there was a significant increase in strength along a much wider strength curve than previously thought. The study showed that there were increases in strength at the angles of +5 degrees, and -5 degrees to the isometric hold position.

More importantly, more extensive studies have subsequently found that with isometric contraction exercises, there is a much wider strength curve benefit than was first thought. The later studies found that between 20% and 50% of strength-transfer occurs at the angles of +20 degrees, and -20 degrees to the isometric hold position. It also concluded that there was a significant increase in strength along a much wider strength curve than previously thought. The study showed that there were increases in strength at the angles of +5 degrees, and -5 degrees to the isometric hold position.

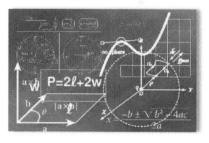

This is huge, and it completely dispels all myths about any potential issues about this. The additional research also concluded that for those athletes who wanted to achieve the most complete and constant curve strength gain, it was comparatively easy to achieve with isometric contraction exercises, especially when compared to regular isotonic weight training.

To achieve the most complete and constant-curve strength gain possible, an advanced athlete would simply perform an isometric contraction exercise at two, three, or perhaps even more positions along the complete range of a joint/muscular range of motion.

To do this properly, it's worth briefly examining how this would work in practice, starting with a recap about biomechanics. A normal, healthy limb has a certain Range

of Motion, AKA: ROM.  This is the arc through which the
movement takes place at a joint, or series of joints.  This

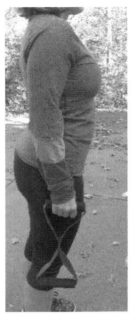 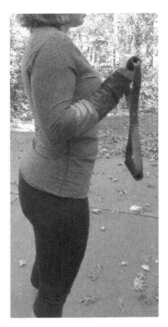

Zero Degrees                    130 Degrees

ROM is technically called "Osteokinematic" motion.

Taking the biceps curl as an example, the range of
motion for that movement in the pictures starts at zero
when the hand is in the lower position and goes up to
approximately 130 degrees in the upper position.

Next, if we assume that there's a strength-curve
benefit of +20 degrees, and -20 degrees around the point at
which an isometric contraction is performed, then we can
calculate the approximate positions to perform the
additional isometric contraction exercises.

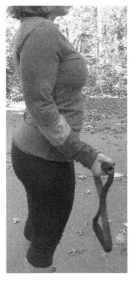

The first position could be at approximately 20 degrees from the neutral starting point because this would give a strength-curve benefit covering the first 40 degrees of the ROM.

20 Degrees

The second position could be at approximately 50 degrees from the starting point because this would safely overlap the first strength-curve arc from about the 30-degree point and extend up to about 70 degrees.

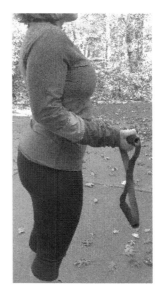

50 Degrees

The last position could be at approximately 80 to 95 degrees from the starting point. This would then overlap the last, from the 60-degree point, and provide a strength-curve benefit across the higher end of the arc, getting closer towards the 130-degree maximum ROM of the limb.

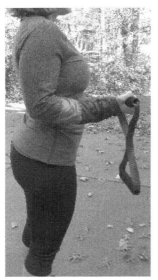

80-95 Degrees

If necessary, a highly advanced athlete might also want to add an additional isometric contraction exercise at the very starting point of the ROM of the limb. This would then strengthen the muscles when in the most mechanically disadvantaged position.

Naturally, for those who are isometric enthusiasts like myself, the information in this

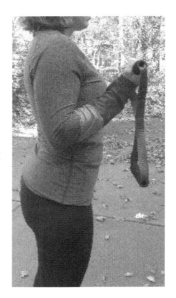

130 Degrees

chapter is very interesting, however, does it relate to The Bullworker 90™ Course in some much deeper way?

## Rest - How Much, and How Often?

There is a direct proportion between the intensity and quantity of exercise, and the amount of recovery time that's needed after it. After all exercise, and especially after

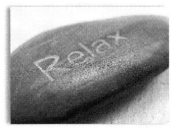

high-intensity exercise, your muscles require a recovery period to repair, recover and grow. This typically takes anything from 24 to 48 hours.

It's also important to remember that your muscles don't grow during your workout, they only really grow after your workout, during the recovery period. Exercising too often will prevent complete recovery from taking place, and it will eventually deplete your muscle tissue and have the completely opposite effect to what you wish to achieve.

When calculating the ideal recovery period, many things should be taking into consideration, all of which are based upon the individual concerned. For some people, this recovery period will need to be longer than between 24 and 48 hours. The recovery period will also need to incrementally increase as the intensity of the exercises increases towards an individual's 100% potential maximum capacity.

For advanced and professional athletes who perform isometric exercises at 100%, or near 100% maximum contraction, the rest and recovery time between exercise sessions becomes much more important. Research has indicated that in this respect, athletes should perform only 3 or 4 workouts per week because of the higher

228

demands being placed upon the Central Nervous System (CNS).

Extensive research about this was performed independently by leading experts: Professor Yuri Verkhoshansky, Professor William J. Kraemer, PhD Human Performance Laboratory, University of Connecticut, and Dr Steven Fleck PhD, Chair of Sports Science, Colorado College and Head of Physical Conditioning Program for the U.S. Olympic Committee.

For the average person who wants to shape-up, tone-up, look better, and to feel better, sports scientist J. Atha's research revealed something remarkable. The research showed that when performing a routine of isometric contraction exercises at only a $2/3^{rd}$'s of an individual's maximum capacity, they could exercise this way daily without any risk of overtraining.

This is excellent news for anyone who wants to use isometric exercise as a means of general strength development, basic body shaping, and even for moderate bodybuilding. Since an ideal workout, which would be suitable for almost everyone, would involve a series of isometric holds at only $2/3^{rd}$'s of their maximum intensity, it's always going to be entirely based upon the individual concerned. It also means that the isometric exercises in the ISOfitness™ system can be safely performed daily by almost anyone, of almost any age, and in almost any physical condition. Naturally, only after approval to exercise this way has first been granted by a doctor.

Other factors which positively affect post-exercise recovery include a balanced and properly executed stretching routine. Getting plenty of quality sleep is also vital, because when you sleep your body releases hormones to help you repair and rebuild damaged tissue, which will directly help your muscles to grow.

High-quality nutrition after a workout will help your body to repair itself faster, improve your post-exercise recovery time, and help to generally maximise the benefits gained from the exercise. There are studies that indicate there is a 30 to 60-minute window of time for eating after exercise before your body begins to draw upon itself to repair and recover from your exercise session.

If time is short, and convenience is a factor, then we recommend a water-based vegan shake such as Raw Fusion. Also, don't forget about drinking lots of water either. This is one of the most important factors in your overall health and fitness routine, your muscles are mostly composed of water, therefore, it's a vitally important factor in post-exercise recovery.

## *The Blood Pressure Myth*

Many people like to point out the fact that when someone performs an isometric exercise it will raise their blood pressure. However, the same people also very conveniently forget that it is also true of all other forms of exercise including freehand callisthenics and traditional isotonic resistance training with weights.

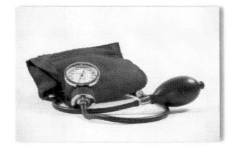

Approximately 20% of the heart's resting output goes to the major muscles of the body. Naturally, during exercise, this level will increase and the blood vessels in your muscles get bigger, or dilate, as the flow of blood increases. This process allows more oxygen to be delivered to the muscle being exercised. Muscular contraction and especially isometric exercises consume large quantities of oxygen. The muscle which is being contracted during exercise needs to be able to greatly increase its blood flow and subsequent oxygen delivery process. This means that changes in muscular resistance and the blood flowing to the muscle being exercised will have a direct impact on your arterial pressure and blood flow. For example, during particularly intense isometric exercise around 80%, or more, of the heart's output goes to the muscle being contracted.

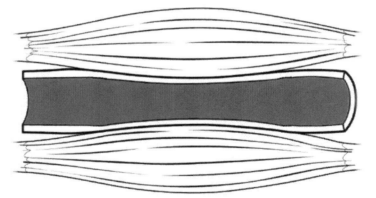

**A very basic representation of a relaxed muscle with a free-flowing artery running through it.**

It's important to remember that when an isometric contraction begins, the blood flow to the muscle being exercised briefly decreases. This is because the muscle which is being contracted applies a direct pressure to the arteries, veins, and overall structure of that muscle, which in turn restricts the blood flowing into it. This is called extravascular compression, and blood flow into the muscle only increases again once the muscles begin to relax. It should be remembered that ALL physical activity, and especially exercise, will cause your blood pressure to rise for a short time. Providing that you are in good health, that you always breathe deeply, naturally, and normally when performing any exercise, then any rise in blood pressure experienced during exercise will soon return to a normal level when the exercise is stopped. The faster this happens, the fitter you are.

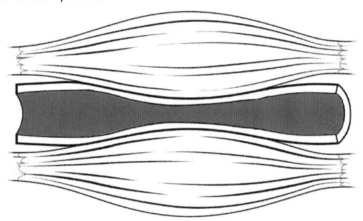

**A very basic representation of a tensed muscle restricting the artery running through it.**

We know from the work of Dr Nicolas Babault PhD in 2001, intramuscular tension lasts an average of about 1/3$^{rd}$ of a second for each isotonic repetition of resistance training. Therefore, we also know that this means there is less venous constriction during each isotonic repetition than there is during an isometric exercise because the latter holds the intramuscular tension much longer. For healthy individuals, this isn't typically a problem. For those who are advanced athletes and/or are used to hard and intense isometric training for a long time, then you'll already have made significant progress in strengthening your heart and circulatory system. For those who are new to isometric training, just like with any form of exercise, the best way into it is by taking it slowly and less intensely at first. Newcomers to exercise, and especially isometrics, should always focus on applying less intensity to begin with, and on always breathing fully a deeply throughout all exercises. NEVER HOLD YOUR BREATH!

Research led by Charles Kivowitz, M.D. and William W. Parmley, M.D., at the Department of Cardiology, Cedars-Sinai Medical Center and the Department of Medicine, University of California at Los Angeles, California, has indicated that for people in normal health, with no heart disease, any rise in blood pressure during isometric exercise is solely because of increased cardiac output, and not because of coronary artery disease.

Research published in the European Journal of Preventive Cardiology Published on Oct 1, 2014, found that Quadriceps Isometric Strength is a predictor of exercise capacity in Coronary Artery Disease patients, and it may be used to set strength training goals according to a patient's needs.

It's just a fact that ALL physical activity, and especially exercise, will cause your blood pressure to rise for a short time. Providing that you are in good health, that you always breathe deeply, naturally, and normally when performing any exercise, then any rise in blood pressure experienced during exercise will soon return to a normal level when the exercise is stopped. The faster this happens, the fitter you are.

Under strict medical supervision, even those with Coronary Artery Disease, and high blood pressure should be able to increase their physical activity levels with a reasonable degree of safety safely. However, if you're a person who already suffers from high blood pressure, then you should always exercise at a much lower level of intensity than someone who has no physical issues. Furthermore, **EVERYONE, AND ESPECIALLY PEOPLE WITH HYPERTENSION, OR ANY FORM OF CARDIOVASCULAR DISEASE, SHOULD ALWAYS CHECK WITH THEIR DOCTOR BEFORE BEGINNING ANY KIND OF EXERCISE ROUTINE**.

It's interesting to note that in 2014 the Mayo Clinic published a report which found that performing regular isometric exercise lowers blood pressure and the resting heart rate. Therefore, it may also help reduce the risk of developing heart disease. This shouldn't be too surprising, because most forms of regular exercise, including isometrics, will have an overall beneficial effect on your blood pressure levels.

## *Why Aren't Isometrics More Popular?*

"If isometric exercises are so good, then why aren't they more popular then?" This is a good question, and there are several reasons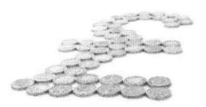

for this. The main answer is very simple: There is much less money to be made commercially out of promoting isometric training, especially when compared to regular isotonic exercises and general weight training. This is one reason why you don't see many supportive editorials about the superiority of isometric exercise in glossy fitness magazines.

Many, and in some cases, all the editorial content in a bodybuilding and fitness magazine is usually some sort of paid-for commercial advertising. There's more money made from advertising other forms of exercise and products than there is out of tyring to sell simple and inexpensive to perform isometrics.

The reality is that to perform a full-body, maximum contraction isometric workout, even an advanced athlete doesn't need to go to an expensive gym. You can't sell a wide range of expensive equipment, because you just don't need it.

If isometric exercises were suddenly as popular as traditional weight training, then commercial fitness clubs wouldn't exist in the way that we know them today. People would be getting all the results they want, faster, easier, and without an expensive gym membership. Furthermore, they'd be getting those results by working out almost anywhere, on almost any location.

For many people, the social aspect of being a member of a fitness club is very important, and we'd strongly encourage that because it can lead to a healthier way of life. Group exercise sessions can be a lot of fun, and it's always nice to make new friends.

For many other people, and we include ourselves in this respect, we want the "biggest bang for our buck." We just want to get the best results we can get from our exercise sessions, we want the exercise sessions to be as brief as necessary to get the job done properly, and we then want to be able to devote the rest of our spare time to doing other things, rather than spending all our spare time exercising.

Another reason why isometric exercise isn't more popular is that some people suffer from a common syndrome. This is that they "confuse activity with accomplishment."

Furthermore, they do this in all aspects of their life, and not just in respect to exercise. For people who confuse activity with accomplishment, it just "feels" like they're achieving more in performing movement-based exercises. People conveniently forget that with all things in life, love, and business, it's never the quantity of what you do that

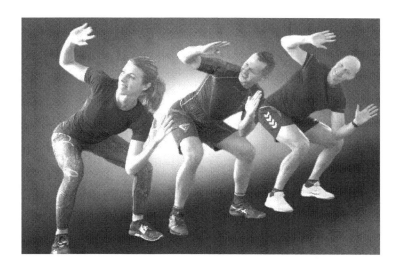

counts, it's always the quality of what you do which will get the best results.

Failure to recognise this crucial point will mean that you can easily waste lots of time, money, energy, and effort in doing things which are at best less efficient, or at worst, completely useless. In exercise terms, many people are a wandering generality, instead of being a meaningful-specific. Isometric exercises are a perfect example of being a meaningful-specific. They are a precisely targeted, scientifically proven, and an extremely efficient way to shape, tone, and build both strength and muscle.

Since people are just much more familiar with movement-based exercises, and it takes quite a lot of convincing to encourage people to even try isometric exercise. However, once people have tried them, and start to get excellent results from exercises which last for only seconds per day, then they're usually "sold" for life on isometric exercise.

Perhaps a static exercise system just isn't as "sexy" as movement-based resistance exercises, or in telling your friends that you train with weights at a gym. Maybe it's just harder to impress others by performing comparatively "quiet" isometrics, instead of literally throwing weights around.

Let's not forget that nothing is "sexy" unless someone, usually who is famous in the media, considers it to be so. It's almost straight out of the short tale "The Emperor's New Clothes" by Hans Christian Andersen, in that something is only "hip" or "sexy" because the masses are sold on it being that way. Very few, if any, will deliberately disagree, despite what their common sense tells them.

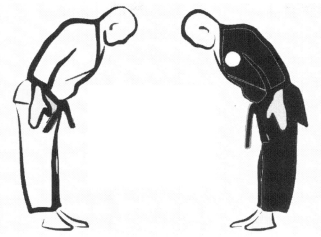

Another important point to remember is that systems like Yoga, and many of the Martial Arts, already use isometric exercises as an integral part of their training system. However, these are usually performed under different names. Fitness coaches either simply don't know enough about the science of isometric exercise, or if they do, they certainly don't want to teach it to their clients. If they do, then they'll very soon need a regular supply of new clients because the existing ones have discovered they don't need an expensive gym and expensive associated coaching fees.

Being "sold" on fun is another important factor why isometrics aren't more popular. Today, there is a proliferation of home-use exercise equipment. These are typically sold via infomercials, and they suddenly make getting into shape seems more like an amusement theme park event, because it's all about fun, right?

Naturally, there's nothing wrong with having fun. However, where's the fun in having to exercise for lengthy periods of time, and often with expensive gadgets that don't get the job done very efficiently, if at all? We've already established that for every home exercise gadget that works, there's always another one being sold which doesn't work and is basically expensive junk.

When performed at a high-intensity level, isometric exercises can be very hard work, and most people are inherently lazy. It takes lots of willpower, and determination, to push yourself to achieve a near maximum contraction during each isometric exercise.

Of course, the great bonus to isometric exercise is that you only should perform each hold for 7 seconds, therefore, when compared to regular weight training exercises, it's all over quickly. Besides this, most people will never need to exceed 2/3$^{rd}$'s of their individual maximum capacity.

## *Functional Strength?*

There's no such thing as non-functional strength. This is because any sort of strength will always be functional to some degree. When critics of any exercise system highlight "it doesn't increase functional strength" as a possible disadvantage, it's a ridiculous statement. All exercise systems that increase strength, don't always prepare someone to use it functionally in every aspect of sports, or life in general. Instead, there are simply different functions of strength and being strong.

Are Olympic weightlifters functionally strong?  They certainly are in the sense they can lift a weight in Olympic style.  When they're in overall strength competitions such as "The World's Strongest Man" contest, they can fail miserably in performing a "farmer's walk," or in overturning a car.

Therefore, in terms of strength, functionality is always going to be subjective.  If you're already strong, then it's going to be easier to develop certain skills to make your strength "functional," and to perform certain things to a high level of ability.  For example, the sport of wrestling requires certain skills to be developed to execute throws, locks and holds to a high level.

For example, a person who simply has great strength who doesn't have those same skills, won't be able to perform the sport of wrestling with any sort of competency.  Someone who has developed exceptional strength and fitness will be able to learn those essential skills and eventually perform them to a high level of competency.

At that point, they'll have both skill-competency and great strength, which will make them a better overall wrestler than if they had only developed the skills alone.  In the words of my old martial arts master, "If two people possess equal skills, the person who is stronger will always win, so always endeavour to become strong as well as skilled."  Being strong will always help you to do whatever you choose to do, better than if you weren't as strong.  It's that simple.

# Chapter 7: A Brief History of Isometric Exercise

By now, you may be wondering how the concept of isometrics all began, so we'll give you a brief history. To do this we could go as far back as several hundred, and possibly even several thousands of years. This long ago, even though they didn't understand any of the science behind it all, people had still learned about how beneficial "static" hold exercises were. The terms "static," and "static hold" have been well referenced in many ancient manuscripts and texts. We'll spare you all that, and instead, we'll begin in more recent history, approximately 100 years ago, with one of the first scientific studies performed about movement-based exercises.

In the 1920s, just after World War 1, scientists at Springfield College in Springfield Massachusetts, USA, were performing experiments to study how long periods of inactivity affected the muscles of bed-ridden injured service veterans from World War 1.

In a now-famous experiment, the scientists wanted to determine how much muscle loss there would be in a limb which was restricted in movement to the point where it was static, in comparison to a limb left free to move and exercise freely. In researching the effects of atrophy, or muscle wasting/shrinkage, on an immobile leg, they conducted a series of tests, using frogs as the initial test subjects.

To do this, they secured one leg of each frog so that it completely immobilized it. This left the remaining leg free to move, and naturally, the frog moved it a great deal as it tried to escape captivity. In doing so, the frog unknowingly "exercised" its free leg by kicking repeatedly, just like in traditional isotonic exercise, as it pushed hard to free itself.

Before the experiment, the scientists involved had all predicted that the outcome of the experiment would be about comparing the varying degrees of atrophy in the immobile leg, to how much growth there would be in the leg which was left free to exercise with movement. The scientists also predicted that the unfettered leg would grow significantly in both muscle size and strength when compared to the immobile leg.

The results of these experiments were completely unexpected, in fact, they were startling, and they had massive long-term ramifications. This is because the results were the opposite of what the scientists had initially predicted. After only two weeks, the immobile leg of all the test frogs had grown significantly stronger, and larger, compared to the leg that had been left free to move as it tried to escape. In fact, the static leg had grown so much stronger and larger than the mobile leg that when the frogs were released, they apparently jumped one-sided due to the muscular size and strength differential.

Little did they know it at the time, but the scientists at Springfield College had made an incredible breakthrough-discovery about comparative performance advantages of isometric contraction exercise, over multiple repetition isotonic exercises. What was perhaps even more amazing than the discoveries they made, was the fact that the team of scientists never applied the new discovery to the rehabilitation of veterans, nor was it applied to sports training.  Amazingly, it was ignored at the time, and very quickly it was almost completely forgotten about.

In 1953, after a gap of almost 30 years, new research studies were commissioned at the world-famous Max Planck Institute in Germany about the science behind isometric contraction exercise.  As we know, this extensive research unfailingly concluded the superiority of isometric contraction exercises when seeking to increase muscle size and strength.  This was the research study that proved repeatedly that a single, daily isometric contraction, held for a period of between only 6 and 7 seconds, and using only $2/3^{rd}$'s of a person's overall maximum capacity, had the ability to increase their strength by up to 5% per week.  Other subsequent studies found very similar test results, and others found even more, with one scientist having documented strength gains in volunteer test subjects improving by an incredible 300%, although this result could never be repeated in further tests.

While researching at the Max Planck Institute in the late 1950s and early 1960s, the famous sportsman, coach,

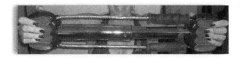 and inventor Gert F. Kölbel, eventually conceived the idea for a new exercise device.

This would be one of the first practical exercise devices based on the "new," and scientifically proven principles of isometric contraction exercise.  Gert F. Kölbel invented a device which he initially called the "Tensolator," and later renamed it as "The Bullworker®."

The rest, as they say, is history. The amazing Bullworker® device fully utilised the principles of isometric contraction exercise in a completely practical way. It enabled the user to perform a comprehensive range of exercises, using the single, and more importantly, a completely adjustment-free device which could easily be used at home.

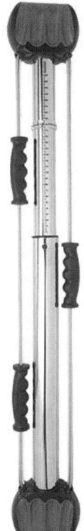

The Bullworker® was an instant hit. Bob Hoffman, who was the coach to the US Olympic weightlifting team, and representative on The President's Council for Physical Fitness, used isometric contraction exercises extremely effectively as part of his coaching system.

The German Olympic weightlifting team also used isometric contraction exercises, and with great success when training for the 1972 Olympic Games.

Thanks mainly to isometrics, their athletes literally "swept" the medal board. Sadly, the appalling terrorist attack on the Israeli athletes dramatically overshadowed all the sporting successes.

On a lighter note, the Bullworker® was so effective and successful that it won the praise and support of many leading celebrity athletes, including, Bruce Lee, Mohamed Ali, Arnold Schwarzenegger, and Dave Prowse. Incidentally, it was Dave Prowse who was the weightlifting champion

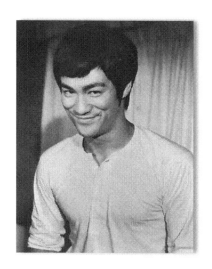

behind the Darth Vader mask in the original Star Wars movies.

The late 1970s was when the use of isometrics began to fall into decline. It did so to make way for the

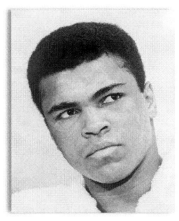

more "sexy" forms of group aerobic exercise dance classes, which also heralded the beginning of the boom in social fitness clubs. These early fitness clubs eventually evolved to become the large commercial brand-name chains we see throughout the western world today. Even though isometric exercises were proven to be extremely effective, they simply weren't considered to be that much fun, and socially acceptable in the new fitness clubs. Besides this, it was

246

always going to be much harder trying to justify high membership fees to have members exercise isometrically with exercises that require little or no equipment.

Eventually, with the aerobics boom generating increasingly massive momentum, isometrics were somehow forgotten about. The huge advertising budgets of the "sexy" new aerobic systems, such as those fronted by celebrities like Jane Fonda, also did a lot to encourage the public to forget about isometrics.

In the mid-'80s, I met, started training with, and I eventually occasionally coached my friend and 4 times World's Strongest Man winner, Jon Pall Sigmarsson of Iceland. Jon Pall told me that he personally believed that it was the isometric exercise system we used that gave him the competitive edge he needed to become one of the strongest men of all time.

Today it's very different. There are now many more people who are interested solely in getting real results from their exercises. They are strong enough emotionally to use an exercise system based on the outstanding results it gives them, and not about how socially acceptable, or commercially "sexy" the system might be. The result is that isometric contraction exercises are now making a steady return to popularity, with more people than ever before discovering and embracing them with an open mind. In addition to this, there are now several new variations of isometric contraction exercise, all of which are based upon, and around, the proven scientific principles. This makes it easier than ever to find an isometric exercise system specifically suited to the goals of an individual.

247

Outstanding isometric-based devices such as the Iso-Bow® and Iso-Gym® are easily affordable and widely available.  Even the Bullworker® is being produced once again and sold all over the world.   When used in combination with the ISOfitness™ system, and "The 70 Second Difference™" concept, it means that even the busiest people can now maintain a highly effective regular workout routine, even when travelling away from home.  Even serious athletes never need to miss a high-quality gym-level workout.  These systems are a huge bonus for everyone who simply wants to get into shape, stay in shape, even if they don't have much spare time.  It's also a huge bonus for anyone who doesn't have a huge budget to spend, and who needs a highly effective exercise system for minimum outlay.

### *NASA and Isometrics*

I've often been asked why NASA hasn't more readily embraced isometric exercises as the preferred method of choice for astronauts.  As one might imagine, NASA has a "natural" interest in isometric exercise because they require little or no equipment for even an advanced workout to be performed.  Therefore, if isometrics could provide a viable exercise solution, it would dramatically reduce the take-off weight of a spacecraft, and free-up some extremely valuable room inside which would otherwise be filled by bulky isotonic resistance exercise equipment.

It's not simply a case of NASA declaring officially about either the effectiveness of isometric exercise when compared to traditional isotonic exercises. The issue is much more serious because the mystery which NASA needs to solve ASAP is about why an anti-gravity environment somehow switches off certain vital functions of the human body. Also, why astronauts still suffer muscle atrophy despite performing all kinds of exercise, and why even the human immune system seems to switch off in space.

In 2018, the results of year-long tests will be published comparing the effects of how space travel in an anti-gravity environment affects the human body. Two identical twin NASA astronauts were the test subjects, with one of the twins, Scott Kelly, living in space on the International Space Station for 340 days, and the other twin, Mark Kelly, living entirely on Earth. This would allow scientists to perform the most detailed comparison study to date.

Preliminary results have been surprising. It revealed that astronaut Scott Kelly's genes suffered hundreds of serious mutations after spending only a year in space. The anti-gravity environment somehow forces the body to turn various immune functions on, and off. Comparisons studies were also made about how space travel affects genes, the gut microbiome, and various aspects of phycological health.

Astronaut Scott Kelly's chromosome caps, or telomeres, physically lengthened while living in space, and then shortened again once he was back on earth. Telomeres prevent our DNA from damage, and naturally shorten as we get older, which is one of the reasons we physically change with age. NASA suspects that these are directly affected by astronaut Kelly's exercise routine, and diet while he was in space. This is one of the reasons why NASA is so keen to determine which are the best kinds of exercises, or exercise systems to perform in an anti-gravity environment.

As you're probably already aware, fast twitch muscle fibres provide the power needed for lifting etc., and slow twitch fibres enable a person to stand upright and perform basic daily functions etc. Both muscle types use the protein myosin as a common building block. This governs how muscle contracts, and with what power. On Earth, under normal gravitational load, the myosin gene remains active. This gene becomes mysteriously inactive when in zero gravity, where no force whatsoever is being produced by the body.

If they don't solve these critically important problems quickly, then unless scientists can develop a simulated gravitational field which can be built into all future spacecraft, at the end of a long space flight astronauts would be physically weak, and possibly very sick too, when they arrive at their destination and experience some sort of gravity again.

Since we already know that the many isotonic resistance exercises that astronauts have been performing for a long time don't work to prevent muscular atrophy, then what are the comparison results between those exercises and roughly equivalent isometric exercises?

To find an answer to these and many other exercise and immune system related problems, NASA commissioned an extensive study. They decided to start at a molecular/chemical level and work upwards from there in examining the basics of why muscle grows, why workout sessions produce results when on Earth, and if isometric exercises are effective at building muscle.

Since the first study took place in 2004, many people in the exercise community have clearly misunderstood it, and completely misinterpreted many of the initial results.

The first study NASA conducted was led by physiology Professor Kenneth Baldwin, from the Department of Physiology and Biophysics at the University of California, Irvine, USA. Professor Baldwin et al set out to compare the benefits of isometric exercises against isotonic concentric AKA lifting/contracting, and isotonic eccentric AKA lowering/lengthening, and then examine the results right down to the chemical level.

This is the point where it all became a little bizarre in my opinion. This is because both the test subjects that were chosen for the study and the choice of "physical exercise," were somewhat curious, to say the least.

Instead of examining some of the many studies which had already been published and using them as a basis of their new study for NASA, amazingly, Professor Baldwin decided not to test humans, and not to use actual physical exercise in their research.

At this point I sat back in my chair in disbelief, and repeated in my inner monologue, "The objective is to study the why exercise works, and the effectiveness of certain exercises on humans, however, they're not going to use humans in their study, and they're not even going to use actual physical exercise, instead they're going to use rats as test subjects and only simulated exercise through electrical stimulus?"

It's common knowledge in the exercise community that a plethora of 1st class research studies have already been completed into the effectiveness of isometric exercise, and how it compares to isotonic resistance training. Furthermore, these studies have been performed by some of the finest exercise scientists who have ever lived, at some of the most prestigious institutions. The first and perhaps the most famous which comes to mind is the 5-year study on 5,500 people of all levels of athletic ability performed by Dr Hettinger and Dr Mueller at the Max Plank Institute in Germany.

Incidentally, in case you're unaware of just how clever the people are at the Max Plank Institute, then search online to see how they landed a space probe on a moving comet travelling at thousands of miles per hour over 4 million miles away. This is the sort of serious research and science that the Max Plank Institute undertakes.

From the thousands of studies conducted into exercise over the decades, we already know the ideal recovery timescale for humans after strenuous exercise, how to generate maximum muscle fibre engagement and the optimum isometric exercise time etc.

Conversely, I'm betting that there's no data anywhere in the world about how long it takes rats to recover from strenuous exercise, and how to best generate maximum muscle fibre engagement in a rat during exercise.

I'm also betting that Dr Hettinger and Dr Mueller at the Max Plank institute somehow forgot to include rats in their 5-year study of isometric exercise.

I'm well aware of the effectiveness of electronic stimulation, and how it is used as a sports training aid. This is in humans, not rats. I also understand why, and how, it is much easier to perform a biopsy of muscle tissue from a rat, rather than from a human.

Yes, I'm being a little sarcastic in some of the paragraphs above, and I'm sure that you can see why that is. Moreover, if you're a taxpayer in the United States, then you may wish to begin questioning what these people spend your hard-earned tax dollars on. In 2004 Professor Baldwin was appointed for 4 years to oversee a program with $2.5 million per year funding, in addition to this, Professor Baldwin and Professor Caiozzo each received $1.5 million in grant money from the National Space Biomedical Research Institute. You can read more about this here on science daily.com: https://www.sciencedaily.com/releases/2004/05/04052505 5749.htm

Setting aside my sarcasm about what NASA spends US taxpayer's money on, the results of the initial study was very encouraging. Even though we know absolutely nothing about how a rat responds to physical exercise, and even though they could naturally only use electric stimulation and not actual physical exercise, the initial study, and subsequent studies, clearly showed that isometric exercise wasn't just the equal of other types of isotonic exercise, it was slightly better.

Now that landing on Mars is officially NASA's next goal, it'll be very interesting to see how these studies progress, and what the results will eventually be. The fact is that we all really need to know why workout sessions work, why we respond to exercise and grow muscle, and how to prevent the human immune system from switching itself off when an astronaut is weightless in space.

I'm especially curious to see if because of the research studies, they choose to use either isometric exercise alone or in combination with other isotonic exercises for astronauts in space. I'm also curious to see if NASA then decides to spend millions of dollars to develop new isometric exercise equipment to use in space when a simple Iso-Bow could probably do the job just as effectively for a fraction of the cost.

## Chapter 8: Isometric Exercise Techniques

Since the time of the ground-breaking research carried out regarding the effectiveness of isometrics by Dr Hettinger and Dr Muller in the 1950s, several other isometric-based styles and techniques have been devised.

Each new technique and concept, extended and expanded, on the basic standard isometric contraction exercise. These new techniques and concepts now mean that isometric-based exercise can be used effectively to not only build great strength and increase muscle size but to also develop greater endurance, improve athletic ability, and for competitive bodybuilding.

Many of the names we use to describe these techniques and concepts may also be familiar under other names because they have become increasingly popular training methods amongst fitness enthusiasts, sports people, and athletes of all types.

## Standard Isometric Contraction

Standard Isometric Contraction, AKA: overcoming isometric contraction, AKA: Maximum-Effort Isometrics, is when a muscle is applying force to push or pull against an immovable resistance. We've already covered the science about this quite extensively, together with some of the background, in earlier sections because this type of isometric contraction exercise was used in the experiments performed by Dr T. Hettinger and Dr E. Muller. It's also the exercise technique referred to in their book "The Physiology of Strength," making it the basis of all other isometric contraction techniques.

In a Standard Isometric Contraction, one can theoretically exert 100% of their maximum capacity effort against an immovable object, and then continue to hold that level of intensity throughout the duration of the exercise. The only real variable is the practitioner's perception of what their 100% maximum effort is. We've already established that the individual's perception of exactly what 100% is will vary between someone who's an experienced professional athlete and an absolute beginner to exercise.

Experience has also taught us that most beginners will always fall well short of even estimating what 2/3$^{rd}$'s of their 100% maximum is. In fact, many might believe they're performing at 100% capacity. If they were tested properly, they might only be performing at about 70% of their overall maximum. Therefore, that's the target we generally encourage our personal coaching clients to aim for.

The immovable object can be an object such as a wall, door jamb, motor vehicle or something similar. The main thing is that it's completely immoveable to human muscle power alone. A specific isometric-based exercise device can also be used and preferred for biomechanical reasons. Perhaps the best, and the most practical are the Iso-Bow®, the Bullworker®, or the Steel Bow®. They can each be used without any adjustment, and with equal effectiveness by a complete beginner, or by an advanced and highly trained sports professional. The benefits received will still be proportionally the same.

In a traditional gym, things like power racks, smith machines, most pin-selector or disc loaded exercise machines, and even barbells and dumbbells can be used. Some coaches may prefer to use things like steel chains and cables, which are adjustable in length and can be anchored

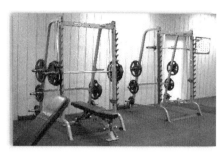 to immovable belay points. Another excellent way is to use self-resistance. This is where one limb or body part, is pitted against an opposing limb or body part.

Self-resistance exercises are an excellent way to ensure that a personal maximum resistance is used safely and with minimum risk of injury caused by applying too much force. The Iso-Bow®, the Bullworker®, and the Steel Bow® are all excellent in this respect. Since it's compact, versatile, and inexpensive, we highly recommend the Iso-Bow® for sheer all-around compact versatility.

The Iso-Bow® has the added advantage in making self-resistance more stable for wrists, elbows, and other joints. The Iso-Bow® a very practical tool which gives you something ergonomically correct to grip, unlike when performing self-resistance exercise hand to hand. This is essential in helping to prevent injury while allowing the user to apply their maximum intensity in each exercise.

According to research performed by Dr Hiroaki Kanehisa in 2002 and Ross Enamait in 2005, the improvement of the torque-to-muscle-volume ratio is more effective in other forms of isometric training than it is in Standard Isometric Contraction. For those of you who don't already know, torque, or movement of force, is the

258

tendency of a force to rotate an object. In this case, it's a joint, body part or limb, around an axis, fulcrum, or pivot point. Whereas force, is a push or a pull, torque can be thought of as being the twist to an object.

A debate continues amongst scientists about the speed at which tension should be applied during an isometric contraction. Our personal preference is to apply the tension over a period of up to 3 or even 4 seconds, before beginning to count the required 7-second hold of the isometric contraction and to reverse the procedure when the exercise is over to disengage.

The research is clear in that when seeking to develop explosive strength and power, it's more effective to produce the tension quickly. Sports science researchers Messrs Fleck and Kramer produced the research about this in 2004. We believe that the risk-to-benefit ratio of injury is too great with this method. This is because it's also proven that the risk of injury is always significantly higher when tension is developed quickly.

## *Yielding Isometric Contraction*

Yielding Isometric Contraction exercise is when a muscle, or muscle group is targeted and set against a resistance which is the desired percentage of an individual's personal maximum capacity. Instead of working to apply force against the immovable object, in yielding isometric exercise, the muscle and joint oppose the resistance provided by the object for as long as possible, or for a set length of time.

Standard Isometric Contraction is a purer isometric contraction as detailed in the experiments of Dr Hettinger and Dr Muller. This is because the practitioner can usually, in theory, always exert even more force as a percentage of their overall maximum capacity against a completely immovable object. Therefore, the direction of the force is always concentric in nature.

In Yielding Isometric Contraction exercise, the resistance force is only slightly concentric in nature, and 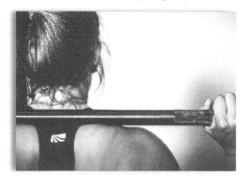 most of the force is always in the eccentric action of resistance during the exercise. The practitioner is always trying to prevent the chosen resistance from forcing the limb into performing an eccentric motion because the whole object of the exercise is to prevent any eccentric motion from taking place. The overall intention is to prevent any form of movement, in either the eccentric or the concentric phase.

When performing Yielding Isometric Contraction exercise to failure, naturally, the limb will ultimately slowly move in the eccentric phase. This might even increase in speed as the ability of the muscles starts to progressively fail in preventing any movement from taking place. The resistance-time usually moves well beyond the 7-second strength building barrier as noted by Dr Hettinger and Dr Muller, taking it into the endurance exercise phase. Using the barbell curl as an example, one would hold the bar at a given position along the range of movement for the exercise, and a precise amount of pressure would be applied by the biceps to neutralise the resistance. The objective is to hold the position, so that the bar is neither lowered, nor lifted higher, and resistance continues to be applied throughout the process of complete muscle failure.

Yielding Isometric Contraction exercise makes it possible to more easily measure progress than in Standard Isometric Contraction exercise. The use of devices like the Bullworker® made the measurement of progress relatively easy in the performance of several different types of isometric contraction exercise. Many coaches also believe that the pressure provided by a "real resistance" is superior in building strength, as opposed to simply using an opposing self-resistance. There is no current scientific data to support this theory. By simple default, the use of heavy weights as resistance in overcoming isometric exercise will also increase the risk of injury.

The famous Canadian strength coach Christian Thibaudeau, perhaps unsurprisingly noted in a 2004 scientific study, that Yielding Isometric Contraction has a greater impact in strength gains, and in increasing muscle mass, when in the eccentric phase. His research also clearly showed that Standard Isometric Contraction naturally has a greater impact on strength gains in the concentric phase. Interestingly, he also noted that they do not have the same effect on a practitioner's neural patterns.

Why is the eccentric phase of an exercise more effective in building strength and muscle size, than it is by exercising in the concentric phase?  During the eccentric part of any resistance training movement, many beneficial things happen including the stimulation and engagement of more muscle fibres, and in especially the fast-twitch fibres, which are the ones that mostly contribute to increased muscular size.  There are increases in neural pathway stimulation, and more microtrauma to the sarcomeres is produced, and in addition to this, the new chemical bonds produced are very strong, which results in longer lasting muscle and strength gains.   When practically using Yielding Isometric Contraction, the training load used should range from between 50 and 80% of the individual's overall maximum capacity, and it should last for a duration of between 30 and 60 seconds.

## *Maximum Duration Isometrics*

Maximum Duration Isometric, AKA: MDI, exercise is when you are applying isometric force by pushing, pulling, or holding a submaximal load for as long as possible.  These are not pure isometric exercises to build strength in the classic sense, however, they are excellent at increasing endurance.  The length of time a Maximum Duration Isometric hold is applied for is usually never to absolute failure, instead, it will range between 30 and 60 seconds in length.

The famous Canadian strength coach Christian Thibaudeau noted in his 2004 scientific study, that this form of training creates a high level of micro muscle damage, and it can be extremely effective in the development of muscle volume.  This makes it an excellent choice for bodybuilders who want to use the isometric exercise system.  It's also possible that this style of isometric training might relate to what is commonly called the sarcoplasmic hypertrophy effect. There is no current data available to confirm or disprove this hypothesis.

## *Explosive Isometrics, AKA: Ballistic Isometrics*

Explosive Isometrics focuses almost entirely on developing isometric tension as quickly as possible. This is then held for very brief bursts of between 1 and 3 seconds, and it's a variation of Standard Isometric Contraction. According to the highly respected Canadian strength coach Christian Thibaudeau, his 2004 scientific research study showed that this method is excellent at developing a balance of both speed and strength. Furthermore, it's often found in practical sporting use when training in the "hard." external styles of martial arts.

Explosive Isometric exercises are excellent at improving the performance of athletes who participate in sports which require that extremely rapid movement should take place from a resting start. This would include sports such as the martial arts, sprinters and other track athletes, shot putters, rugby players, American football players, and in Olympic weightlifting.

The research that was performed by famous sports scientists P. D. Olson and W. G. Hopkins in 1999 was to determine practical examples of how explosive isometric training can be of benefit in various sports, and could significantly increase peak force and speed.

Famous sports scientist D.G. Behm, of Memorial University of Newfoundland, Canada, and D.G. Sale published in 1993 "Intended Rather than Actual Movement Velocity Determines Velocity Specific Training Response." In that excellent work, they found that repeated attempts to perform explosive isometric contractions, with a high rate of force and tension, were the primary stimuli needed for effective high-velocity training response to be produced. The results of their work also supported some similar research, which I was involved in at Manchester Metropolitan University about the effects of speed and neuromuscular reaction time. The conclusions drawn by Messers D.G. Behm and D.G. Sale was that it was the **intention** to move fast, rather than the actual speed of movement which was more important. Once again, the power of the mind and belief is a vital factor in all aspects of life, and sport. We personally believe that the risk to benefit ratio of injury is just too great with this method, especially for the non-professional athlete.

## *Static-Dynamic Isometrics*

Static-Dynamic Isometrics involve supersets of both isometric and dynamic exercises, with minimum or no rest between them. At the start of training, an isometric hold lasting between 3 and 6 seconds is performed, and this is then followed by an explosive dynamic exercise. A good example of this would be pressing the bar of a Smith Machine in the bench press exercise. The bar would be secured by the Smith Machine's pins, to make it immovable.

264

After a predetermined time of between 3 and 6 seconds, the isotonic bench press movement would then immediately be performed. In 1977, Professor Yuri Verkhoshansky's research clearly showed that the combination of the static isometric-dynamic method of training was up to 20% more effective in developing speed and strength when compared to dynamic training alone.

## Dynamic Flexation™

The Dynamic Flexation™ technique is a form of static-dynamic isometric exercise, which incorporates elements of other isometric techniques including yielding, maximum duration, overcoming, and standard isometric contraction.

Dynamic Flexation™ involves performing extremely slow and precisely executed exercise movement throughout the Range of Motion of a limb to fully engage the muscles in every isometric exercise. To some degree, everyone will employ a basic form of Dynamic Flexation™ as they find the correct position and begin to engage their muscles before exercising them.

Even for a beginner, we would always recommend that to some degree everyone employs a form of Dynamic Flexation™. This will help to ensure that all muscles, tendons, ligaments, joints, and spine become naturally and properly engaged in the correct isometric exercise position, which will usually be helped by taking a correct hand grip, fist clench, or foot position.

This means that you should always ensure that you perform each exercise in the correct biomechanical position to gain maximum benefit from each exercise. When you assume the correct position, to begin with, you should apply almost no tension whatsoever.

Instead, you should "feel" your way into ensuring that you're in the correct position *before* beginning to apply tension to the exercise. Once you're in the correct position, perhaps the worst thing to do would be to suddenly apply maximum tension and at the same time hold your breath. This is completely wrong. Remember to always breathe naturally as you gradually engage your muscles into the exercise.

Our personal preference is to apply the tension gradually through Dynamic Flexation™, over a period of up to 3 or even 4 seconds. This is before beginning to count the required 7-second exercise hold of the isometric contraction.

During the exercise, be sure to breathe naturally and deeply. We prefer using each full breath in and out as a method of counting more accurately the number of seconds each exercise is performed, with one breath in and out representing one second.

Similarly, at the end of an exercise, we don't recommend that it be ended abruptly. We prefer to reverse the Dynamic Flexation™ technique, and to gradually relax and slightly move each muscle and joint as you do so. Here's a diagram which explains the workflow visually.

| Dynamic Flexation™ 2 to 3 Seconds | 7 Second Isometric Exercise | Dynamic Flexation™ 2 to 3 Seconds |
|---|---|---|

Dynamic Flexation™ is a concept which embraces the broader principles of motor unit recruitment, and "Henneman's Size Principle," to increase the contractile strength of a muscle. Elwood Henneman's principle stated that, under load, the motor units in a muscle are engaged according to their magnitude of force output, from the smallest to the largest, and in task-appropriate order.

This means that the slow-twitch, low-force, fatigue-resistant muscle fibres are activated before any fast-twitch, high-force muscle fibres are engaged which are less fatigue-resistant. Since the body works in this way, it enables precise, finely controlled force to be delivered at all levels of output. This also means that when exercising, or when performing tasks in daily life, the fatigue which is experienced as a result will be always be minimised, and proportional to the sequential engagement of the most appropriate muscle fibres.

There are limitations as to what beginners should expect to be able to do. It's important that no one should ever perform exercises or techniques beyond what they're capable of performing safely and effectively. The advanced Dynamic Flexation™ techniques are something we'd only recommend for intermediate, advanced, professional athletes.

Advanced Dynamic Flexation™ involves slowly engaging the muscles you're about to exercise, and then introducing only a very slight movement of Dynamic Flexation™ in the concentric, and eccentric planes of motion for as many as 10 repetitions before fully engaging the muscles in the Standard Isometric Contraction exercise. The Dynamic Flexation™ technique should always be performed slowly in both directions, in accordance with your natural breathing pattern, and to help create the maximum muscular engagement at the end of it.

For those who wish to create a greater muscle pump effect for pure bodybuilding purposes, then we suggest increasing the Dynamic Flexation™ movement should be performed as suggested above. It should also be performed with an even greater range of motion in both directions, to complete a full range of movement in the exercise. If you're in any doubt about the speed of motion when performing Dynamic Flexation™, then as a rule, always perform the technique slower. Since the performance of Dynamic Flexation™ technique is typically able to be off-set by self-resistance, or other forms of resistance, it allows the opportunity for someone focussed on bodybuilding to develop the maximum muscle pump possible, in just one pre-, and/or post-isometric contraction set.

When the Dynamic Flexation™ technique is performed properly, it should almost completely neutralise the strength and power of the opposing muscle group to such a degree that a single Dynamic Flexation™ repetition takes several seconds to perform in each direction, while still employing almost maximum muscular intensity and engagement.

As you might imagine, when it's performed correctly, this technique is demanding. Therefore, we suggest that it should only be used by advanced and professional athletes. It places an extraordinary demand upon the cardiovascular system, the muscles being directly exercised, the supporting and core musculature, and the CNS, or Central Nervous System.

When incorporating this level of Dynamic Flexation™ technique into an exercise routine, it will result in the rest and recovery time between each workout session being almost certainly extended. If it isn't, then overtraining may becoming an issue.

We can't stress strongly enough the importance of only, and always performing all forms of exercise and especially any sort of Dynamic Flexation™ pre-isometric engagement movement, with excellent exercise styles and absolute precision. Once you've completed your chosen type of pre-isometric engagement Dynamic Flexation™ technique, then when you finally do engage the muscles, make sure that you always engage them as close to the desired level of intensity as possible.

Dynamic Flexation™ also incorporates aspects of what we call "functional isokinetic exercise." This is because this is an applied, practical workout technique which is all about the force that a muscle applies during the movement of a limb while at a constant velocity.

### The Iso-Bow® Difference

The Iso-Bow® is a product we fully endorse and highly recommend. It's inexpensive, high quality, and it works exceptionally well. An amazing Iso-Bow® costs

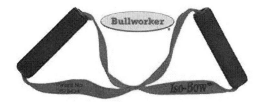

"pennies" in comparison to other exercise devices, and even a pair of them can easily fit into your pocket, they never need adjusting, they can deliver a total-body workout at the perfect level of intensity for either a complete unfit beginner or an advanced athlete.

We're not even endorsing our own products, we're simply endorsing a product which we believe will be the best investment you'll ever make if you want to get fit, strong, and in the best shape of your life.

The company that makes the Iso-Bow® is Hughes Marketing LLC, and they also produce a small range of other high equally exercise products, which

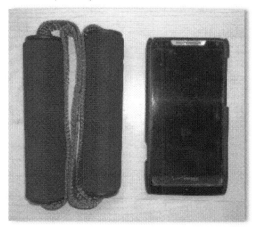

all deliver excellent results at a fair price.

Brian has personally used nothing more than a pair of Iso-Bows® as the base of his entire body shaping and

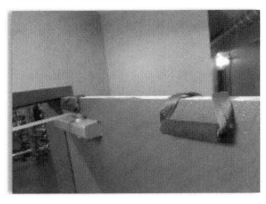

fitness routine for several years now.

Therefore, we know that the Iso-Bow® is "the real deal," and it delivers exceptionally good results. Helen incorporated the Iso-Bow® into her own workout routine, and she believes that it was the Iso-Bow® that made the difference and enabled her to win the 1st place prize in her last Bikini Fitness competition.

The Iso-Bow® is versatile too, and it can be used with equal effectiveness as both an isotonic, and an isometric exercise device. It allows the user to perform highly-effective self-resisted isotonic exercises for almost every muscle group.

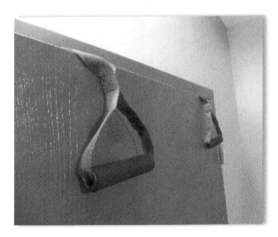

A pair of Iso-Bows® can even be used as a great doorway pull-up device,

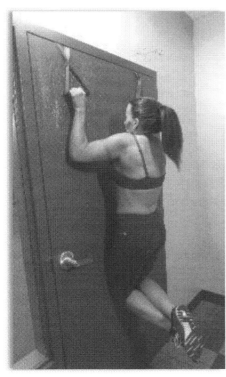

which can even fold up and slip right into your pocket when you're done. Try doing that with a regular, clumsy steel doorway pull-up bar.

The Iso-Bow® is naturally a first-class isometric exercise device, and it allows a very wide range of exercises to be performed that work almost every muscle group of the body. It also allows the effective execution of more advanced techniques to be performed within the ISOfitness™ system.

Since the Iso-Bow® is so inexpensive, well designed, well-constructed, and extremely useful in ways we haven't even begun to describe here in this book, it's not so much a recommendation for you to get a pair, rather an instruction for you to do so. We

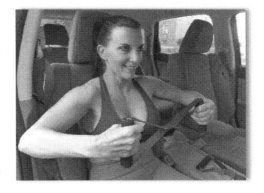

believe that you'll soon see why these inexpensive devices are what we believe to be the finest, most versatile, and most powerful of all exercise devices which have ever been invented. That's a bold statement, but it's made from our heart, and it's delivered with our most sincere belief in the product and how you will benefit from owning a pair, and in using them correctly. Don't forget, we don't make this product, we simply believe in it to that degree of commitment.

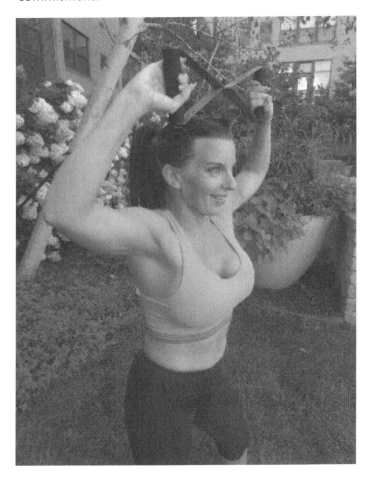

## Chapter 9: The 70 Second Difference™ Workout

The exercises in "The 70 Second Difference™" workout have been specially selected so that all the major

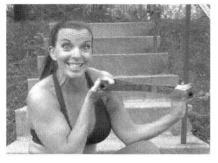

muscle groups will be exercised effectively in just 70 seconds of continuous exercise time.

In addition, these exercises will help to ensure that your core muscles are engaged as much as possible, and your Base Metabolic Rate is stimulated, to kick-start the fat burning process while you're building muscle at the same time.

The exercises contained in "The 70 Second Difference™" workout can be performed by anyone, at any level, from absolute beginner, right up to the professional athlete. This is because all exercises and workout routines in the ISOfitness™ system, work with your natural Adaptive Response™ mechanism. Therefore, the results you get are entirely dependent upon the level of focus, effort, intensity, you apply to each exercise.

If you're already at an advanced level of fitness and strength, then you can naturally exert more effort and intensity into each exercise. In doing so, you will engage more muscle fibres in the process. Even though there are only 7 exercises to perform, if you apply close to 100% of your maximum effort, then even if you're a professional athlete, you'll still gain the benefit from even a simple 7 high-intensity exercise session.

The ISOfitness™ system offers the user something that isn't possible with any other common exercise system. This is the ability to perform a professional standard high-level workout, almost anywhere, and in a fraction of the time of a traditional workout. This makes the ISOfitness™ exercise system, and "The 70 Second Difference™" workout ideal, even for advanced and professional athletes when they're travelling away from home either on business or holiday. Even if life just somehow gets in the way, and there doesn't seem to be enough hours in a day, then with "The 70 Second Difference™" workout, you are always able to maintain a basic but effective exercise routine.

## *Always Get Medical Approval*

Everyone, no matter what level of fitness they're at, or how long you have been exercising regularly for, you should always get medical approval from your personal physician before beginning this, or any other kind of exercise or diet system.

It's always a good idea to show your physician the complete workout routines, exercise techniques, and diet

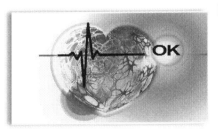 plans you intend to perform. That way they'll have a complete understanding of what you will be doing. They'll then be able to make an informed decision about whether they recommend that you proceed, or not. Only once you have received the full approval from your physician, should you then begin any exercise routine.

Never strain or push yourself beyond your safe physical limits during any exercise. If at any time you feel light-headed, faint, or show any other sign of having a potential issue, then stop exercising immediately and consult your physician.

## *Securing the Iso-Bow® With Your Feet*

When performing leg exercises such as squats and lunges, as well as lower back and glute exercises such as deadlift, it

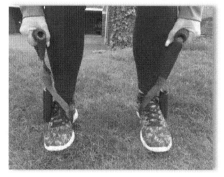

becomes necessary to properly secure the Iso-Bow® using your feet.

There are several ways in which the Iso-Bow® can be secured using your feet, and your personal preference of how you do this will depend upon many factors such as your foot size, your choice of footwear, and ease of operation.

You can secure the Iso-Bow® with your foot inside one of the handles. You do this by adjusting the handgrip to one side, usually the

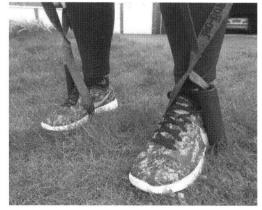

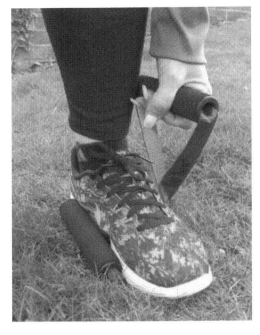

outer side of the foot, and then place your feet inside the loop like a stirrup.

Another method is to place the Iso-Bow® flat on the floor and then stand on one side of the straps so that the handle of the same side sits flush to your inner foot. In this position, it will be your bodyweight combined with the handle pressing against

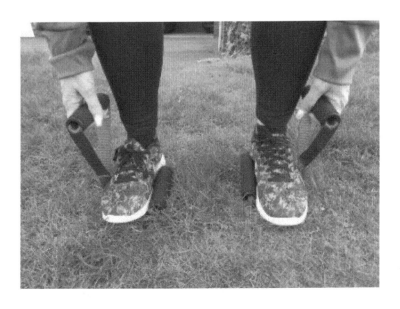

the inner side of your foot which enables you pull safely and securely.

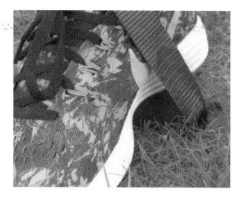

The final method is to simply place each foot through one end of an Iso-Bow®, stepping onto the foam hand grip as you do so. This

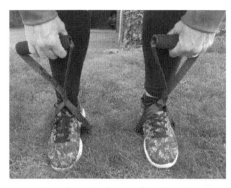

method offers slightly less stability than the other two methods. However, if the foot can be pushed far enough through the loop of the Iso-Bow® handle, then the handle will slightly raise the level of your heel making it easier for some people to squat or lunge.

Naturally, safety is always a top priority so whichever method you ultimately choose to use, you should always make sure that when securing the Iso-Bow® with your feet that there is never any

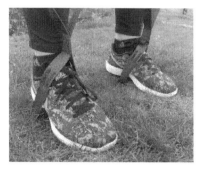

chance of it slipping in any way while you exercise.

### *Shortening the Iso-Bow® - The Cradle*

Generally, the Iso-Bow® is the ideal size for most users, and for most exercises. However, occasionally you may prefer to reduce its operational size by roughly half, by creating what we call an Iso-Bow® cradle.

To do this you place one of the handles inside the webbing loop of the other handle side of the device. The handle you've just placed inside the loop is then cradled by the webbing and can be gripped as normal. Your thumb, and fingers can then wrap around both the foam handle and the webbing of the cradle-loop to help ensure an even firmer grip position is created.

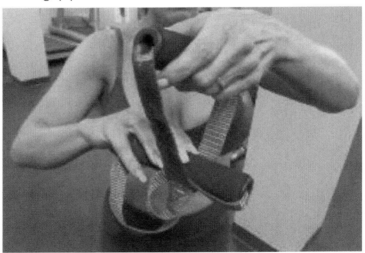

This reduced size allows for an even greater operational range within the movement capability of each limb/joint to be created for certain exercises. These include The Cross-Chest Press, The Upper Back Power Pull, and The Biceps and Triceps Cradle Press-Curl.

279

## *Before You Begin - Recapping the Basics*

⚠ The first and perhaps the most important thing to remember is: **NEVER HOLD YOUR BREATH AT ANY TIME, AND EACH DEEP BREATH WILL COUNT THE NUMBER OF SECONDS IN EACH EXERCISE**.

⚠ Breathing in and out naturally during all isometric exercises will also help you count the number of elapsed seconds much more accurately.

⚠ We recommend that you read the instructions about each workout routine and exercise carefully. You can also watch the associated videos on the ISOfitness™ website.

⚠ Weight loss/fat loss will ONLY occur when ISOfitness™ exercises, or ANY other exercise plan, is used in conjunction with a calorie-controlled diet.

⚠ It's critically important to completely focus your mind on the exercise being performed, and in addition to this, to fully envision the muscle growing and getting stronger.

⚠ Always consult a professional coach to devise a detailed stretching routine, this will ensure that you're stretching the areas effectively rather than risking injury. Always ensure that a stable line of biomechanical progression is achieved before engaging in and performing any exercise.

⚠ Warming-up, stretching, and cooling down are three of the most overlooked, yet essential elements to exercise, and we cannot stress their importance strongly enough. During ANY form of physical exercise, including isometrics, if you apply too much intensity too soon, then you may inadvertently strain a muscle. Isometric exercise is particularly intense, and a single isometric exercise engages a great many more muscle fibres than even high-intensity weight training, and isometrics engages the muscle fibres at a much higher level too.

**For safety's sake, we're adamant that you should always gradually and progressively engage your muscles into ANY isometric exercise, and according to what we call The ISOfitness™ Exercise Timeline.**

The main benefit to properly warming up for several minutes before a workout is injury prevention, and to increase your heart rate and the circulation to your muscles, ligaments and tendons. It's important to remember that warming-up and stretching are two different concepts and stretching isn't a good warm-up. This is because stretching will put the muscle in an un-contracted position and weaken it. Stretching is always best performed after a workout has been completed, together with a proper cool-down.

In addition to properly warming-up, always perform a gentle "flex and stretch" of the muscles and joints which are about to be exercised. For example, squatting down fully to flex the thighs and loosen the knees is always a good idea before performing any leg exercises. Dynamic Flexation™ should always be used with every ISOfitness™ style isometric exercise. Here's a diagram which explains the workflow visually.

| Dynamic Flexation™ 2 to 3 Seconds | **7 Second Isometric Exercise** | Dynamic Flexation™ 2 to 3 Seconds |
|---|---|---|

ISOfitness™ style isometric exercises are deceptively powerful. Even when engaging in what may feel like only moderate intensity exercise, you're probably still engaging and contracting a great many more muscle fibres than you would in a similar isotonic exercise. If you're in any doubt whatsoever, then always perform the exercise with a little less intensity. In addition to a proper warm-up, the Dynamic Flexation™, performed in conjunction with the isometric exercise, will help to ensure a greater blood supply to the muscles and surrounding tissue.

**ALL ISOfitness™ exercises and workout plans work equally well for men AND women. BOTH sexes can build great strength, solid muscle, body build, or simply get into great shape if they wish, each according to their natural potential.**

It's just a fact that consistency is always going to be the key to success in any exercise routine. One of the biggest mistakes people make when exercising is to let their workout routine grow stale. At that point, they're simply going through the motion when exercising and falling way short of deriving maximum benefit for their efforts. By making sure that you always perform some sort of balanced exercise routine on a regular basis, no matter what happens around your life, is always going to produce the best results. This is the way to gain the maximum benefits from isometrics to make you strong and build more muscle. One of the great strengths of isometrics is that they can probably be performed a wider variety of ways than any other type of exercise regimen. This fact will certainly help everyone maintain a consistent routine. As a general rule, always change your routine every two or three weeks, or sooner if needed. Mix it all up and try performing some of the more unusual exercises because this will help to keep it all fresh, fun, and results-producing.

Just because Helen Renée usually demonstrates the exercises in our printed products, stills pictures, and in the videos on the members-side of the ISOfitness™ website, it doesn't mean that the exercises and products are only for women. They're NOT! The science, the exercises, the techniques, and the workout routines, all work equally well for both sexes at every level. They work for a complete beginner right up to a sports professional, a serious bodybuilder, and professional strength athlete. Men who think that they need to see a picture of a man exercising in a book to make it a workout routine for men need to get over it and get into the 21st century. Anything else is "dinosaur" thinking!

The exercises in the next chapter are merely suggestions. As are the number of exercise positions demonstrated. You may wish to substitute some of your own which you might prefer. The choice is yours so long as they're biomechanically valid ways to exercise the muscle/s you're targeting. *Finally, please read, review, and ensure that you've fully complied with all recommendations in the section entitled: 'Important General Safety and Health Guidelines,' and only start ISOfitness™ exercises with the full approval of your physician.*

## The Beginner 70-Second Difference Workout
### Legs: Beginner Wall Squat

Target areas and benefits: Front thighs, buttocks, overall

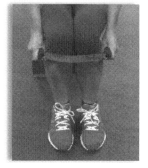

legs, and metabolism booster.

Stand upright, close to a wall, door, vehicle or any other immovable object, to aid with your stability and to help maintain perfect exercise form.

Bend the knees deeply, bending your torso only at the hips, keep your back straight and upright always, and place the Iso-Bow® comfortably around your upper shins as shown. In the wall squat position, grip each handle firmly, and then attempt to stand up straight by engaging the upper thigh and glute muscles. Naturally, you won't be able to move but attempt to maintain a perfect mid-squat position always during the exercise.

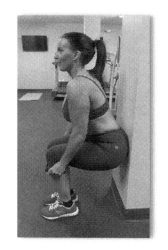

Hold this position as you apply a suitable level of intensity according to your level of ability and breathe naturally and deeply in and out for about 10 full breaths, which will take about 1 second per breath. Aim to perform an exercise breathing count of no less than 7 seconds, and for no longer than 10 seconds.

### Lower Back: Beginner Deadlift

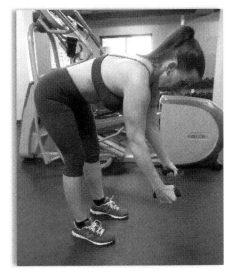

Target areas and benefits: Lower back, buttocks, hamstrings, overall legs, and metabolism booster.

Stand with your feet shoulder width apart, and with your knees slightly bent.

Bend forwards only from the hips as low as you're comfortably able to, hold both handles of an Iso-Bow® downwards towards the floor.

Hold this position as you apply a suitable level of intensity according to your level of ability, and if you want to make the exercise a little more advanced, simply raise your arms forwards.

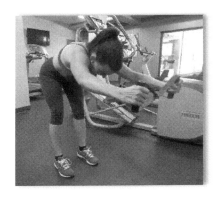

Breathe naturally and deeply in and out for about 10 full breaths, which will take about 1 second per breath. Aim to perform an exercise breathing count of no less than 7 seconds, and for no longer than 10 seconds.

285

## Chest: Cross Press Wide

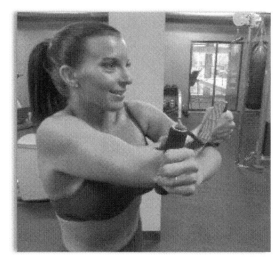

Target areas and benefits: Chest, front shoulders, and overall arms.

Cross the Iso-Bow® in front of you at chest level, with your arms roughly parallel to the floor, and push in opposing directions sideways to engage your chest muscles.

Hold this position as you apply a suitable level of intensity according to your level of ability and breathe naturally and

deeply in and out for about 10 full breaths, which will take about 1 second per breath. Aim to perform an exercise breathing count of no less than 7 seconds, and for no longer than 10 seconds.

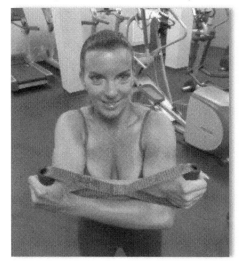

## Arms: Biceps and Triceps

Target areas and benefits: Front and rear upper arms (biceps and triceps), forearms, and front shoulders.

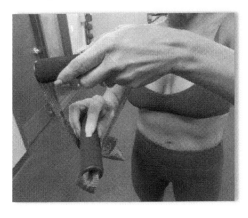

Cradle the Iso-Bow® by placing one handle into the webbing loop-end of the other half of the Iso-Bow®. This is like placing one handle into the cradle of webbing of the other end of the Iso-Bow®. This shortens the Iso-Bow®,

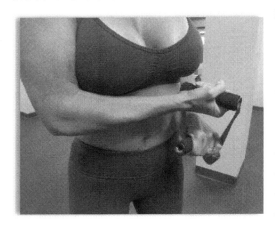

making it roughly half their original size. Cradle the Iso-Bow® with your left hand, gripping the top with your right hand facing up. Grip the cradled side of the Iso-Bow® with the left hand facing down.

Keep both elbows close to your body, and with your right arm across the front of you at waist height. In this position, press down with the left hand, and at the same

287

time press up with the right, to engage both the Biceps and Triceps muscles simultaneously.

Breathe naturally and deeply in and out for about 10 full breaths, which will take about 1 second per breath. Aim to perform an exercise breathing count of no less than 7 seconds, and for no longer than 10 seconds.  Repeat the same exercise for the other arm.

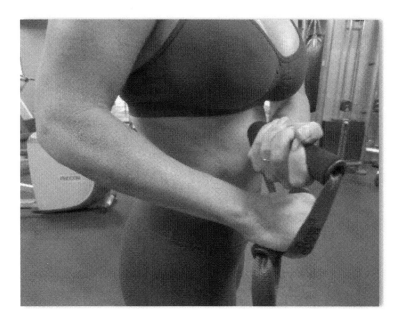

### Back: Seated Single Knee Row

Target areas and benefits: Upper back, rear shoulders, lower back, buttocks, and overall arms.

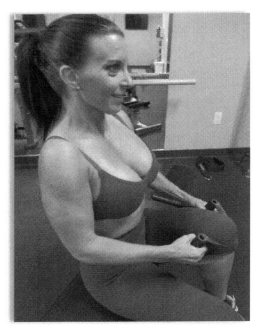

Sit upright on a solid object such as a chair, car seat or bench, bending forwards only from the hips, and keeping your back straight always.

Lift one knee and comfortably wrap the Iso-Bow® around in front of it, pull back with the handles as you engage your upper back muscles, keeping your elbows close to your body as you do so.

Hold this position as you apply a suitable level of intensity according to your level of ability and breathe naturally and deeply in and out for about 10 full breaths, which will take about 1 second per breath.

Aim to perform an exercise breathing count of no less than 7 seconds, and for no longer than 10 seconds.

## *Abdominals: Seated Knee Raise*

Target areas and benefits: Abdominals, core muscles of the upper body, and overall arms.

Place one foot on something stable, a chair, rock, or a bench etc. Hold each end of the Iso-

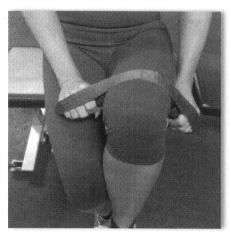

Bow® with a firm grip, with your body upright, place the Iso-Bow® webbing across the thigh, near the knee, of the leg which is bent because it's placed on the raised object.

Keep the Iso-Bow® grips face downwards. Then, slowly engage the abdominal muscles, together with the core muscles of the upper body by curling your body forwards from the hips as you do so. You're attempting to use your abdominals to perform a downward curling motion, a sort of reverse floor trunk curl.

Naturally, you won't be able to do this, nor will you be able to push your raised leg away because it's securely placed on the raised object. As you do so, you will engage your abdominal muscles. Hold this position as you apply a suitable level of intensity according to your level of ability and breathe naturally and deeply in and out for about 10 full breaths, which will take about 1 second per breath. Aim to perform an exercise breathing count of no less than 7 seconds, and for no longer than 10 seconds.

290

## The Intermediate 70-Second Difference Workout

**Note:** If you're at an intermediate level of strength and fitness, then be sure to apply more intensity in each exercise than in the basic level workout.

### Legs: Intermediate Squat

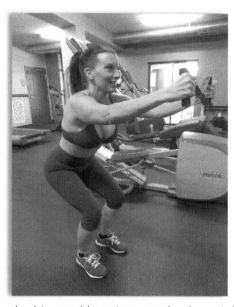

Target areas and benefits: Front thighs, buttocks, overall legs, and metabolism booster.

To perform the intermediate Iso-Squat stand with your feet shoulder width apart.

Bend your knees as far as you're comfortably able to, bending only from the hips and keeping your back straight. Hold both handles of an Iso-Bow® and extend your arms straight out in front of you to aid your balance.

Hold this position as you apply a suitable level of intensity according to your level of ability and breathe naturally and deeply in and out for about 10 full breaths, which will take about 1 second per breath. Aim to perform an exercise breathing count of no less than 7 seconds, and for no longer than 10 seconds.

## Lower Back: Intermediate Deadlift

Target areas and benefits: Lower back, buttocks, hamstrings, overall legs, and metabolism booster.

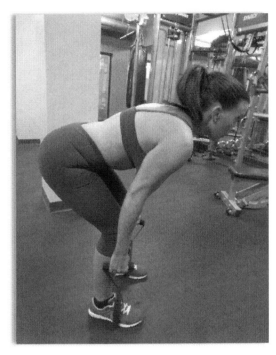

Stand with your feet shoulder width apart, and with your knees slightly bent.

Bend forwards only from the hips as low as you're comfortably able to, hold both handles of an Iso-Bow® downwards towards the floor.

In this position extend your arms and hold the Iso-Bow® straight out in front of you as far as you're comfortable to aid both your balance and to increase the resistance on your lower back muscles.

Hold this position as you apply a suitable level of intensity according to your level of ability and breathe naturally and deeply in and out for about 10 full breaths, which will take about 1 second per breath.

Aim to perform an exercise breathing count of no less than 7 seconds, and for no longer than 10 seconds.

## Chest: Cross Press Wide

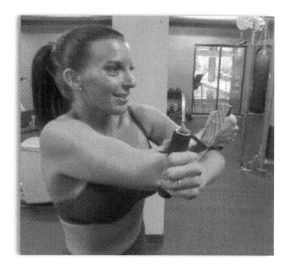

Target areas and benefits: Chest, front shoulders, and overall arms.

Cross the Iso-Bow® in front of you at chest level, with your arms roughly parallel to the floor, and push in opposing directions sideways to engage your chest muscles.

Hold this position as you apply a suitable level of intensity according to your level of ability and breathe naturally and deeply in and out for about 10 full breaths, which will take about 1 second per breath. Aim to perform an exercise breathing count of no less than 7 seconds, and for no longer than 10 seconds.

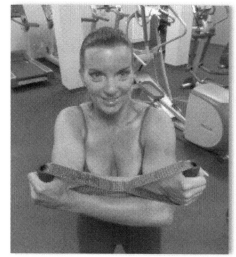

### Arms: Biceps and Triceps

Target areas and benefits: Front and rear upper arms (biceps and triceps), forearms, and front shoulders.

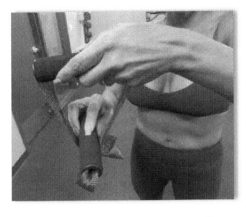

Cradle the Iso-Bow® by placing one handle into the webbing loop-end of the other half of the Iso-Bow®. This is like placing one handle into the cradle of webbing of the other end of the Iso-Bow®. This shortens the Iso-Bow®,

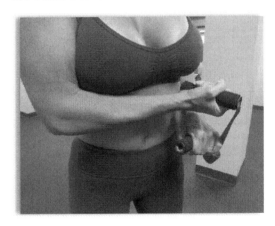

making it roughly half their original size. Cradle the Iso-Bow® with your left hand, gripping the top with your right hand facing up. Grip the cradled side of the Iso-Bow® with the left hand facing down.

Keep both elbows close to your body, and with your right arm across the front of you at waist height. In this position, press down with the left hand, and at the same time press up with the right, to engage both the Biceps and Triceps muscles simultaneously.

Breathe naturally and deeply in and out for about 10 full breaths, which will take about 1 second per breath. Aim to perform an exercise breathing count of no less than 7 seconds, and for no longer than 10 seconds. Repeat the same exercise for the other arm.

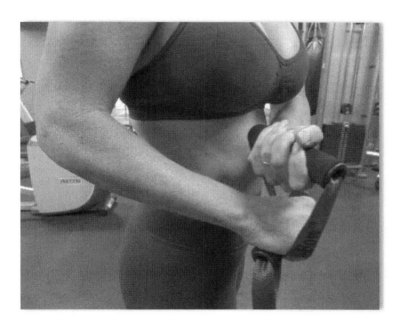

### Back: Seated Single Knee Row

Target areas and benefits: Upper back, rear shoulders, lower back, buttocks, and overall arms.

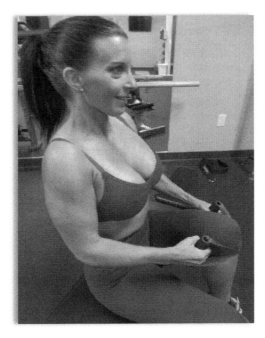

Sit upright on a solid object such as a chair, car seat or bench, bending forwards only from the hips, and keeping your back straight always.

Lift one knee and comfortably wrap the Iso-Bow® around in front of it, pull back with the handles as you engage your upper back muscles, keeping your elbows close to your body as you do so.

Hold this position as you apply a suitable level of intensity according to your level of ability and breathe naturally and deeply in and out for about 10 full breaths, which will take about 1 second per breath.

Aim to perform an exercise breathing count of no less than 7 seconds, and for no longer than 10 seconds.

## Abdominals: Seated Knee Raise

Target areas and benefits: Abdominals, core muscles of the upper body, and overall arms.

Place one foot on something stable, a chair, rock, or a bench etc. Hold each end of the Iso-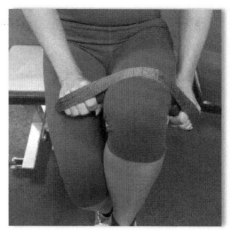
Bow® with a firm grip, with your body upright, place the Iso-Bow® webbing across the thigh, near the knee, of the leg which is bent because it's placed on the raised object.

Keep the Iso-Bow® grips face downwards. Then, slowly engage the abdominal muscles, together with the core muscles of the upper body by curling your body forwards from the hips as you do so. You're attempting to use your abdominals to perform a downward curling motion, a sort of reverse floor trunk curl.

Naturally, you won't be able to do this, nor will you be able to push your raised leg away because it's securely placed on the raised object. However, as you do so, you will engage your abdominal muscles. Hold this position as you apply a suitable level of intensity according to your level of ability and breathe naturally and deeply in and out for about 10 full breaths, which will take about 1 second per breath. Aim to perform an exercise breathing count of no less than 7 seconds, and for no longer than 10 seconds.

## The Advanced 70-Second Difference Workout

**Note:** If you're at an advanced level of strength and fitness, then you should automatically be able to target an appropriate level of intensity for each exercise.

### *Legs: Dual Bow Stirrup Squat*

Target areas and benefits: Front thighs, buttocks, overall legs, and metabolism booster.

Place the looped handle

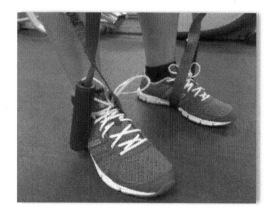

side of each Iso-Bow® around each foot as shown.

Bend your knees deeply to assume the squat position, bending your torso only at the hips, and keeping your back straight and upright always. Grip each Iso-Bow® handle firmly and attempt to stand up straight by engaging your upper thigh and glute muscles.

Naturally, you won't be able to move but continue your attempt to stand up, while maintaining the perfect mid-squat position as you do so. Hold this position as you apply a suitable level of intensity according to your level of ability and breathe naturally and deeply in and out for about 10 full breaths, which will take about 1 second per breath.

Aim to perform an exercise breathing count of no less than 7 seconds, and for no longer than 10 seconds. This

Iso-Bow® stirrup squat exercise is great for the
cardiovascular system and as an overall calorie burner.

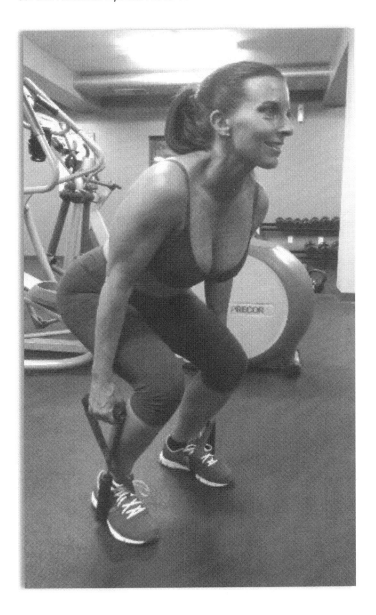

## Lower Back: Straight Leg Deadlift

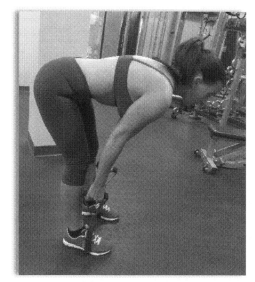

Target areas and benefits: Lower back, buttocks, hamstrings, overall legs, and metabolism booster.

Place the loop handle of both Iso-Bows® around each foot as shown.

Grip the handles firmly, bending over from the hips, with your knees only very slightly bent, and your back straight always, then slowly attempt to stand up straight.

Engage the muscles of the glutes, hamstrings, lower back, thighs, and other core muscles, while the Iso-Bows® secured by your feet prevent any movement from taking place.

Hold this position as you apply a suitable level of intensity according to your level of ability and breathe naturally and deeply in and out for about 10 full breaths, which will take about 1 second per breath.

Aim to perform an exercise breathing count of no less than 7 seconds, and for no longer than 10 seconds. This Iso-Bow® deadlift exercise is great for the cardiovascular system and as an overall calorie burner.

### Chest: Cross Press Cradle

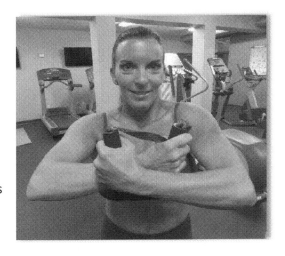

Target areas and benefits: Chest, front shoulders, and overall arms.

Take hold of each handle in across-arms and hands grip position. In this position, you'll be holding the Iso-Bow® in an opposing way across the chest.

Make sure that you hold your arms and elbows at upper-chest and shoulder level and keep the elbows in line with your wrists and shoulders. In this position slowly push each Iso-Bow® further across the chest, naturally, you won't be able to do this, but as you attempt to do so you'll engage the chest muscles.

Hold this position as you apply a suitable level of intensity according to your level of ability and breathe naturally and deeply in and out for about 10 full breaths, which will take about 1 second per breath. Aim to perform an exercise breathing count of no less than 7 seconds, and for no longer than 10 seconds.

303

### *Arms: Biceps Dual Bow Stirrup Curl*

Target areas and benefits: Front upper arms (biceps), forearms, rear upper arm if using your opposite hand as a brace on the thigh, and front shoulders

Lean against a solid object, or sit on a chair, car seat or bench, and place the looped ends of two Iso-Bows® around one foot. Raise that leg slightly until you assume the arm curl position, and then use your leg to provide opposing immovable resistance for your biceps muscles.

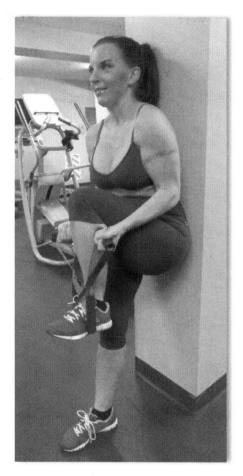

Hold this position as you apply a suitable level of intensity according to your level of ability and breathe naturally and deeply in and out for about 10 full breaths, which will take about 1 second per breath. Aim to perform an exercise breathing count of no less than 7 seconds, and for no longer than 10 seconds.

### *Arms: Triceps Downwards Knee Press*

Target areas and benefits: Rear upper arms (triceps), forearms, and front shoulders

Put one foot on a solid object such as a bench or a chair, or kneel on the floor with one knee extended and place the Iso-Bow® in a comfortable position face downwards, close to the knee and hold both handles.

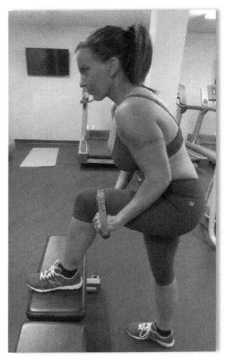

Bend the arms and lean forwards over the knee, and keeping your elbows close to your body always, while pushing down on each handle to engage the triceps muscles of both arms as you attempt to push your body back into an upright position. You won't be able to move, because your bodyweight and your upper body muscles will prevent you.

Hold this position as you apply a suitable level of intensity according to your level of ability and breathe naturally and deeply in and out for about 10 full breaths, which will take about 1 second per breath. Aim to perform an exercise breathing count of no less than 7 seconds, and for no longer than 10 seconds.

## Upper Back: Seated Dual Bow Stirrup Row

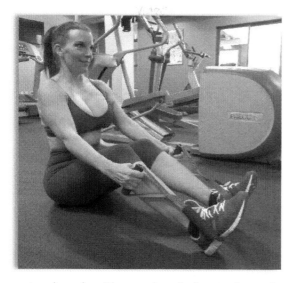

Target areas exercised: upper back, rear shoulders, lower back, overall arms, and glutes.

Sit upright on the floor, or on a chair, car seat or bench with your legs in front of you, bending your knees and hips, keeping the back straight always. Place the one looped end of each Iso-Bow® around each foot, hold the handles firmly and pull your elbows and arms back to engage your upper back muscles, being sure to keep your elbows close to your body as you do so.

Hold this position as you apply a suitable level of intensity according to your level of ability and breathe naturally and deeply in and out for about 10 full breaths, which will take about 1 second per breath. Aim to perform an exercise breathing count of no less than 7 seconds, and for no longer than 10 seconds

### *Abdominals: Foot Supported Trunk Curl*

Target areas and benefits: Abdominals, core muscles of the upper body, and overall arms.

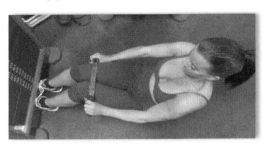

Lay on the floor and place the Iso-Bow® comfortably across the top of the knees. If necessary, place your feet under a solid object that won't tip over to aid both your balance and to allow you to focus more on your abdominal muscles.

Raise your shoulders and body upwards by curling your spine, while at the same time resisting and then preventing

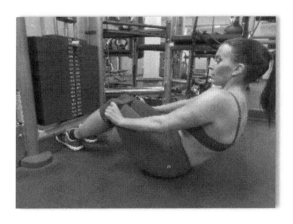

the movement by pressing back on the Iso-Bow®. Hold this position as you apply a suitable level of intensity according to your level of ability and breathe naturally and deeply in and out for about 10 full breaths, which will take about 1 second per breath. Aim to perform an exercise breathing count of no less than 7 seconds, and for no longer than 10 seconds.

## *Chapter 10: Conclusion*

One of the secrets to success in all things, and especially in body shaping and bodybuilding, is regularity in working out. Being consistent in your exercise regimen will help to ensure that you will make rapid and excellent progress towards your desired goals. This has been a real problem for many people because when travelling away from home you're not guaranteed to find a good gym, and traditional home exercise equipment is simply too bulky to carry. With the ISOfitness™ system you can easily replace your gym-confined workout sessions with exercises and workout routines which give you better results and in less time. Anyone who is away from home either on business, or even on holiday, and yet still wants to stay in shape, then they can do exactly that with the ISOfitness™ system. Everyone can benefit from a targeted, intense, and high-quality workout which is completed in only 70 seconds of continuous exercise time. No other workout plan or exercise system is so flexible, works for every level of user, and takes so little time to complete.

Another, more advanced course in the ISOfitness™ system is "The ISO90™" workout. This is a complete 90-day/12-week body shaping, and/or bodybuilding and strength training course. For users who are focused on bodybuilding and strength training, different additional techniques will be incorporated above and beyond those used by the user who simply wants to get into great shape. The ISO90™ course is a step-by-step, week-by-week, month-by-month guide to take you from where you are now, to where you want to be at the end of just 90 days.

Perhaps the most challenging of all our workouts, even for serious fitness athletes, is "The 1664 Workout™."

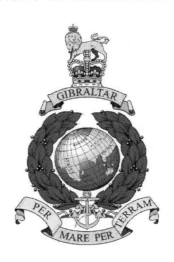

In fact, in our opinion, this is one of the most demanding workout challenges which you'll ever face. It was inspired by the British Royal Marines Commandos, who were founded in 1664, and with 32 weeks of basic training, they officially undergo the longest and most demanding regimen in the world. "The 1664 Workout™" consists of 16 exercises which must be performed at absolute maximum intensity, yet with a target total of only 64 seconds rest time between all exercises. This leaves approximately only 4 seconds between each exercise.

Since "The 1664 Workout™" so challenging, the ISOfitness™ team have even devised a workout challenge to find who the world record holder is for performing the workout at maximum intensity, in the fastest possible time. The workout challenge system is taken directly from my experience gained in winning a Guinness World Record. It has an approved system of how to perform the workout, and for approved adjudication to ensure that it was properly completed according to the rules.   More information about this, and who holds the current record, will be available on both the ISOfitness.uk and helenrenee.uk websites

Every workout in the ISOfitness™ system is available in a similarly comprehensive and complete format.  They're all supported by valuable resource materials including exercise planning charts, food tracking guides and charts, food value calculators, and more as the system grows.  Central to the entire ISOfitness™ workout is video.  Video is one of the most powerful communication tools available

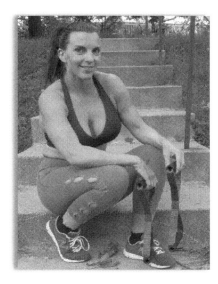

today.  Since at the time of writing, we've already shot over 140 different exercise clips complete with detailed voice and written instruction, it now means that it's possible for our members to create literally hundreds of different workout combinations to tackle any target they might have in fitness, weight loss, sports training, body shaping or bodybuilding.  These new videos will be released at regular intervals, together with other new workout routines and support material. This is the highly practical approach we've taken in making the ISOfitness™ exercise system widely available to all.

No matter what workout or exercise combination you choose to perform in the ISOfitness™ system, they'll always deliver the excellent results you've always wanted. Since no other exercise system works any faster or is more effective, you'll be able to feel the results you get from your very first workout. Within only 5 days of performing the exercises in "The 70 Second Difference™" workout, you'll even begin to see the results unfolding before your eyes.

The fact is that conventional, and out-dated thinking about exercise has been completely challenged by new scientific discoveries about what kind of exercise is best, how exercise should be performed, and how much time should be spent exercising. The scientific conclusions fly directly in the face of everything that many experts had once thought to be constant about exercise. More importantly, these new scientific discoveries completely support and verify the efficacy and power of the exercises, and science behind the ISOfitness™ system.

No one knows what the future holds. However, in respect of exercise, fitness, sports, bodybuilding, and strength training, there finally seems to be a new and infinitely better perspective and level developing which we hope will continue.

Back in the '50s, 60s, and '70s, exercise was very much focussed more on results-based exercise systems which delivered great benefits in terms of overall health, wellness, fitness, and strength. This was a much more open-minded era, when concepts such as isometric exercise were embraced, and employed as part of people's overall routines in the spirit of exploring "new," and scientifically proven results-based systems.  This was one reason why practical isometric/isotonic devices such as The Bullworker® were launched and then became so incredibly successful worldwide.

The Bullworker® almost certainly began the global interest in the proven benefits of isometric exercise.  What also probably helped was that global superstars including Bruce Lee and Muhammad Ali were avid users of The Bullworker®, and they openly endorsed both the device and the isometric exercise system.  What later generations of fitness and sports enthusiasts somehow forgot, was that the superstars who used, recommended, and endorsed isometric exercise, and devices such as The Bullworker®, did so because isometric contraction exercises are the "real deal," they really worked.

Of all the revered superstars who spent their lives in the quest of achieving ultimate fitness, perhaps Bruce Lee was the most famous.  Bruce Lee's strength, fitness, and martial arts ability was legendary, he was a phenomenon and an icon who would go on to influence countless generations in the pursuit of physical perfection.  In respect of his so-called exercise "secret," and how he built his amazing strength, he was completely open about it.  Bruce Lee completely believed in, fully endorsed, extolled the benefits of, and practised daily isometric exercise.

With the dawn of the "aerobic era," something changed which led people away from methods of exercise and solutions which simply "work," and over to a more social aspect of predominately fun-based "wiggle your arse" type of exercise systems, branding, and commercialism.

312

People seemed to become increasingly focused on how they looked while they were exercising, how much fun it was to have a workout, and if their chosen method of exercise was "sexy" and in vogue. They were almost completely disinterested in getting maximum results in the fastest time possible. This shift in perspective lasted a long time, and it's now been several decades since the change began at dawn of the 1980s. In some ways, the emphasis on fun-based exercise and increasingly silly exercise gadgets has increased in infomercial advertising.

In the mid part of the second decade of the 21$^{st}$ century, a re-alignment movement has begun to appear with an increasing number of people began popping up on our "exercise radar" who are more focused on the results they get from an exercise routine, as opposed to how "sexy" or in vogue the routine might be at the time. It's been a refreshing phenomenon to observe, and it continues to grow, even amid the plethora of confusing, and usually useless, exercise and diet systems which big-business always seems to focus on. Why should big business genuinely care if their "solutions" don't really work? Let's face it, they may, in fact, prefer it if their solutions didn't work, because that way consumers will keep coming back for more in the hope that the next glittery offering will be the magic bullet they've been continually promised.

The ISOfitness™ exercise and workout system, which includes "The 70 Second Difference™" workout is all about delivering a solution which is practical, easy enough for virtually anyone to perform, and one which is focussed entirely on the scientifically proven results it can deliver. Do we offer the answer to everything? Do we offer a great panacea? No, of course not. It would be ridiculous for anyone, and for any system to suggest as much. What we do offer has real substance, it has masses of scientific data and proof to show that it works exceptionally well. It also offers you, the open-minded person who has read this book right up to the end, a system of exercise which is inexpensive and extremely effective.

We sincerely wish you every success in whatever your goals in life, love, or business might be.

**The ISOmetric Bible™ - Exercise Anywhere with Scientifically Proven Isometrics**

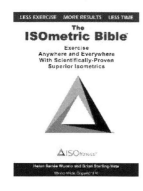

At 335 pages, the ISOmetric Bible™ is one of the most complete, scientific, practical, and user-friendly books on isometrics that's ever been written. Isometrics have been proven by science to grow muscle and strength faster and more efficiently than any other exercise system. It doesn't matter if you're a complete beginner, someone who's already active but wants to do more, or if you're an advanced professional athlete, everyone gets the same proportional benefits to the effort they put in. No time to exercise? Travelling away from home? Are you too busy with work commitments? With isometrics you can exercise your entire body in only minutes each day, they set you free to exercise anywhere and everywhere you choose, on a plane, in a car, or even while you're at work. You don't need any special equipment to get a great total-body workout, but the book shows you how to use easy to find everyday objects such as walking poles, broom handles, rope and towels to exercise with. Exercise science expert Brian Sterling-Vete is a veteran exercise and strength coach and is acclaimed as one of the world's leading authorities on isometrics. Brian has trained multiple national and world champions including 2 x World Martial Arts Champion Stuart Hurst, and 4 x Times World's Strongest Man Jon Pall Sigmarsson of Iceland.

## TRISOmetrics™ - Advanced Science-Based High-Intensity Strength and Muscle Building

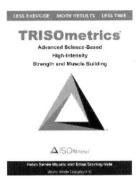

TRISOmetrics™ is an advanced, high-intensity science-based exercise system which combines 3 proven exercise techniques into one powerful workout.  The TRISOmetric™ exercise system will deliver maximum strength gains and muscle growth in minimum time.  Multi-angle isometric contractions provide maximum strength gains through a smooth strength curve along the complete range of motion of a limb.  Maximum muscle fibre engagement is achieved through super-slow isotonic compound combinations, and rest and recovery time optimisation during each exercise delivers outstanding powerful results.  By focussing on precision quality and high-intensity exercise instead of a mediocre quantity means that your workout sessions are kept short in length, infrequent in number, and big on results.  TRISOmetrics™ is part of the ISOfitness™ exercise system and can be used without any special equipment, with the amazing Iso-Bow® exerciser, the Bullworker®, the Steel Bow®, the Bow Extension®, the Iso-Gym®, or any other exercise system you want.  It's also ideal to use with freehand callisthenics and traditional resistance training equipment.  The choice is yours.  The ISOfitness™ exercise system aims to deliver more results, in less time, and with less exercise than any other exercise system.

317

### The ISO90™ Course

ISO90™ is a comprehensive and complete step by step 90-

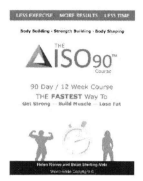

day/12-week body shaping, bodybuilding and functional strength building course based on the ISOfitness™ system of isometric exercises. The ISO90™ course is ideal for beginners, advanced trainers alike. Your natural Adaptive Response™ mechanism means that whatever intensity you apply at whatever level you're at gives everyone roughly the same percentage of improvement. The ISO90™ course focusses the appliance of science in practical exercise and functional strength building, and in doing so, it makes the ISO90™ 90-day/12-week course, one of the fastest, and most efficient ways to get into shape, build muscle, and get strong which has ever been devised. The ISO90™ course allows you to benefit from a professional-level workout literally anywhere and on almost any location. Each week will build upon the gains made in previous weeks, with clear instruction and pictures to

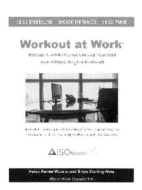

demonstrate how each exercise should be performed. Required Equipment: 2 x Iso-Bows® - available on Amazon or from Bullworker.com

### Workout at Work™

A stark new warning from the Icahn School of Medicine at Mount Sinai School of Medicine in New York reveals that sitting at a desk working for more than 6 hours a day can cause potentially irreversible damage can be done to your heart, together with increases in both cholesterol and body fat, as well as insulin resistance which is a precursor to type 2 diabetes. Even exercising 4 evenings a week after work, or for long periods over the weekend, won't fix the damage. The average person spends over 10 years of their life at work over an average 45 year working life, which can mean sitting at a desk for 10-years! There is never enough time to spare in modern life and exercising the traditional way in a gym 3-days a week, will consume a further 4.27 years. Therefore, time is the #1 reason why people don't exercise. What if you could workout effectively while you were at work? What if a complete beginner could exercise with equal ease to an advanced athlete and all without leaving your desk? Now you can do exactly that with The ISOfitness™ system of advanced isometric exercises. Even if you perform just one 7-second high-intensity exercise every 30 minutes at your desk, you'll gain maximum benefit from this scientifically proven system. At the end of a 9-hour working day you can easily perform an 18-20 exercise total-body workout leaving you healthier, fitter, stronger, and with more time to spend with family and friends. Your boss won't complain either, because in exchange for just 126 seconds out of your working day, you'll be up to 30% more efficient at your job, and you'll take less time off sick. Required Equipment: 2 x Iso-Bows® - available on Amazon or from Bullworker.com

## Fitness on the Move™

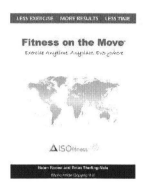

Being able to exercise anywhere is the key to getting the most from your workouts because you'll never be confined to a gym. No matter where you are, or if you're away from home for business or pleasure, you can still maintain a workout to suit all levels of fitness from beginner right up to the advanced professional athlete. The advanced isometric exercises of the ISOfitness™ system have been scientifically proven in over 5,500 independent experiments to be superior to traditional exercise methods. We've tried and tested the Fitness on the Move™ system by performing full workout routines as passengers in cars, on trains, in cramped airline seats, on mountainsides, on beaches, and once even on the deck of a ship in a storm. The ISOfitness™ system of Fitness on the Move™ allows a full-body workout in the smallest space humanly possible thanks to our Zero Footprint Workout™ concept. Required Equipment: 2 x Iso-Bows® - available on Amazon or from Bullworker.com

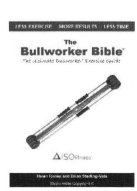

### The Bullworker Bible™

The Bullworker Bible™ is the definitive resource guide for all Bullworker® users, and it's the companion book for The Bullworker 90™ Course. The Bullworker Bible™ is approved by the makers, and distributors of The Bullworker®, at Bullworker.com and it's the complete

320

science-based user-friendly guide of how the Bullworker® should be used properly to deliver maximum results. It also shows you how to effectively use the Bow Extension® and the Steel Bow®. It gives you all the information that you always wanted to know, but the simple wall charts and basic instruction manuals didn't provide. It tells you about Essential Repetition-Compression & Speed Control, Correct Breathing Techniques, Hooke's Law of Physics and The Bullworker®, and Correct Biomechanics for Best Results. The Bullworker Bible™ is also the essential guide for all users of the Bullworker X5, Bully Extreme, ISO 7x, and the Bullworker X7. Required Equipment: A Bullworker® Classic, or a similar device. Recommended Additional Equipment: Steel Bow®, Bow Extension® kit, 2 x Iso-Bows®.

### The Bullworker 90™ Course

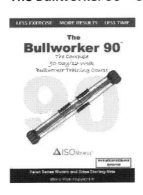

The Bullworker 90™ Course is the essential 90-day/12-week course for all Bullworker® users, and it's the companion book to The Bullworker Bible, approved by the makers, and distributors of The Bullworker®. The Bullworker 90™ is a 400+ page, science-based, user-friendly, step-by-step course designed to increase strength, fitness, grow muscle, body-build, and increase power over a 90-day/12-week period. New exercises are added almost every week, with complete routine changes every two weeks. Each week has a detailed note section, together with suggestions about exercise days, and rest times etc., so that you know exactly what to do, and when to do it. It includes Step-by-step, week-by-

321

week instruction, progressively increasing intensity over 90 days, routine changes every two weeks, isotonic and Isometric exercise combinations, multi-angle isometric exercise combinations. The Bullworker 90™ Course can be used with the Bullworker® Classic, the Steel Bow®, the Bullworker X5, the Bully Extreme, the ISO 7x, and the Bullworker X7. The Bullworker 90™ Course also contains alternative/extra exercises which incorporate the use of the Iso-Bow®, and the Bow Extension® to increase the range and effectiveness of the device. Required Equipment: A Bullworker® Classic, or a similar device. Recommended Equipment: Steel Bow®, Bow Extension® kit, 2 x Iso-Bows®.

**The Doorway to Strength - *Turn a Door into a Strength-Building Multigym.***

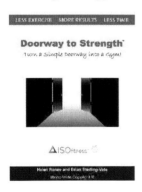

The Doorway to Strength™ shows how a simple door, doorway, and doorframe can be used to create a multi gym of exercises using the amazing Iso-Bow® exerciser and the ISOfitness™ exercise system. It demonstrates how to perform a host of powerful and effective exercises such as the door leg press and shoulder power push, together with many other exercises to work all the major body parts. The Iso-Bow® exerciser is probably the world's smallest and most powerful portable total-body exerciser. They are so small and compact even that a pair of Iso-Bows® can easily fit into the pocket of an average pair of jeans. However, just one Iso-Bow® can deliver the perfect level of workout intensity for a beginner or an advanced athlete, and with no

322

adjustment necessary. The ISOfitness™ exercise system aims to deliver more results, in less time, and with less exercise than any other exercise system. Required Extra Equipment: 2 x Iso-Bows® (preferably 4), a solid door wedge/stop.

## The SSASS™ Course

The Sixty Second ASS Workout™, or SSASS™ workout, is the fastest and most effective "ass" workout ever devised. Based on the scientifically proven principles of the ISOfitness™ exercise system, the SSASS™ workout is a no-nonsense, no time-wasting workout that really does do everything you need to make your ass, tight, firm, shapely, and strong. The SSASS™ routine means no more time-wasting workouts where you twist, shake, wiggle around, kick your legs, or dance around for 30 minutes, which might feel like fun but don't deliver the results you want. Everyone has 60 seconds of time to spare, even on the busiest day, so, you're Just 60 seconds a day from having a great ass. Required Equipment: 2 x Iso-Bows - available on Amazon or from Bullworker.com

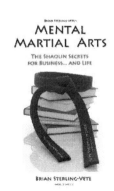

## Mental Martial Arts

Brian Sterling-Vete's Mental Martial Arts is a system of intellectual life-combat skills which uses the tactics and principles of the physical martial arts. All interaction in life, at work and communicating with others is an exchange of energy, power and influence. One party is always

323

exerting maximum influence over the other as they attempt to gain the outcome they prefer over the weaker party. The more powerful and persuasive will usually end as the winner unless the apparently "weaker" person is trained in the martial arts... With this system, you can learn to verbally, intellectually, and emotionally guide, channel, and redirect the energy of others, even more powerful people and large organisations. In doing so, you achieve the outcome you desire in both life and business. It also contains a specific section about how to handle a potentially hostile media in the event of a crisis. Brian combines his system of Mental Martial Arts, together with the experience he gained in over a decade with BBC TV News, to help you and your organisation stay "Media Safe". www.mentalmartialarts.tv

**Tuxedo Warriors**

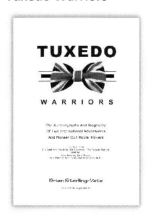

Tuxedo Warriors is the companion book to The Tuxedo Warrior book and movie, which are the autobiography of author, composer, movie-maker Cliff Twemlow. The original book ended at the beginning of what has been called the Golden Age of Video Cinematography, which he inspired. The Tuxedo Warriors is the most complete biography of Cliff Twemlow ever written. It's also the autobiography Brian Sterling-Vete, who played a central role in this unique, entertaining, and true story of two extraordinary "Renaissance-Men" and their adventures as guerrilla movie-makers. They also encountered a poltergeist when living in Iceland, and a UFO encounter which the Police also witnessed. Tuxedo Warriors continues the story where the original book ends. Brian is perhaps the only person who can tell the complete story from the time it all began, right through until the end, with sudden and untimely death of his great friend Cliff.

**The Tuxedo Warrior** by Cliff Twemlow – Prologue and epilogue by Brian Sterling-Vete

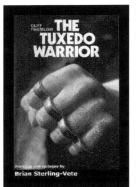

There are many ways in which a Doorman can gain respect. Numerous methods applied to the principal. In my profession, every available technique must be utilised, depending on the situation and circumstances. Would-be transgressors either move-off the premises quietly acknowledging your diplomatic approach. Or, the other alternative whereby physical persuasion must be exercised, which either quells their pugilistic desires, or it triggers their aggressive instincts, turning the whole incident into a bloody and violent encounter. 'The Tuxedo Warrior,' pulls no punches in its brawling, savage, colourful, and entertaining exposure of society's nightlife activities.

The above is the original text from the rear cover of Cliff's book. Cliff and I were extremely close friends, and I'm honoured to re-publish his original work, which completes the storyline of my own book, 'Tuxedo Warriors.' Where Cliff's original book ends, my own book overlaps and

325

begins, to complete his colourful life story. I'm also honoured to be close friends with his eldest son, Barry Twemlow, and sincerely thank him for enabling this book, and others that Cliff wrote, to be re-published.

**The Pike** by Cliff Twemlow – Prologue and epilogue by Brian Sterling-Vete

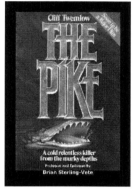

ITS FIRST VICTIMS - A screeching swan... A fisherman overboard... A drunken woman...

One by one, the mysterious killer in Lake Windermere claims its terrified victims. Tearing off limbs with its monstrous teeth, horribly mutilating bodies. Fear sweeps the peaceful holiday resort when experts identify the creature as a giant pike.... A hellish creature with the strength to rupture boats, and the anger to attack them. But for some, the terror becomes a bonanza—the traders who cater to the gathering crowds of ghouls on the shore. And, they will do anything to stop divers finding the creature. Meanwhile the ripples of bloodshed widen.... The Pike

The above is the original text from the rear cover of Cliff's book. I remember this book going into pre-production as a major movie in the early 1980's starring Joan Collins. Sadly, the financiers ran into personal difficulties and it was never made. Today, there is now renewed interest in this book as a screenplay and movie. In my own book, 'Tuxedo Warriors,' I tell the behind the scenes story of myself, my close friend Cliff Twemlow, and The Pike.

**The Beast of Kane** by Cliff Twemlow – Prologue and epilogue by Brian Sterling-Vete

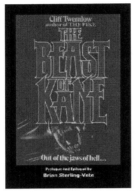

When the Gordon Family open their door to a stray Elkhound, they unwittingly welcome-in the forces of evil. For, according to the local priest, the huge dog is Satan himself, fulfilling an ancient prophecy.

But, no one will believe this warning... Even when sheep – and wolves – are mysteriously slaughtered. Even when frenzied pets turn on their owners. Even when Emily Forrest is savagely eaten alive – the first of many human victims.

As winter tightens its icy grip on the remote town of Kane, its unprotected people must face an unearthly terror.

The above is the original text from the rear cover of Cliff's book. This was the first of Cliff's books to be accepted by Hammer Film Studios to be made into a big-screen horror movie, along with Cliff's other book, The Pike. More importantly, the reason why it was never to be made into a movie was no reflection on the book itself. It was entirely because of the increasing financial challenges Hammer Films were facing at that time. They were issues that were so serious, that they caused the unexpected and rapid decline of the studio.

## Paranormal Investigation - The Black Book of Scientific Ghost Hunting and How to Investigate Paranormal Phenomena

Paranormal Investigation, and especially Ghost Hunting, has long been regarded as a pseudoscience and

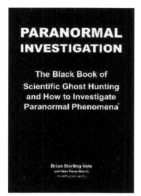

dismissed by closed-minded members of the traditional scientific community. We believe they're wrong to take this approach. Just because they currently can't detect paranormal phenomena in a laboratory, doesn't mean that it doesn't exist.

This book is an objective look at paranormal investigation. it outlines a solid scientific approach that can be used by all paranormal investigators in their research. It also contains several example stories of previously untold paranormal events which have taken place, a ground-breaking UFO sighting, and paranormally active haunted locations. It is ideal for those who are new to paranormal investigation and ghost hunting, and for more experienced investigators who want to learn more about how to apply a critical-path scientific approach. It contains a special scientific critical path graphic page to work from when devising ghost hunting experiments and to help train team members. The book also contains a step-by-step guide to a complete paranormal investigation and important information about how to protect yourself from malevolent paranormal entities that can attack you.

## The Haunting of Lilford Hall - The Birthplace of the United States as a Nation Haunted by the Man Behind The Pilgrim Fathers

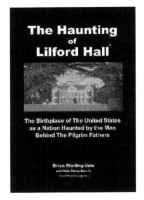

The Haunting of Lilford Hall is one of the most baffling cases of paranormal activity experienced simultaneously by multiple people ever recorded. Between 2012 and 2013, a team of 13 people came together to produce a historical TV documentary, not a paranormal investigation.

The TV documentary was about the life of Robert Browne, the man who was behind The Pilgrim Fathers sailing on The Mayflower to settle the first civilian colony on the American continent and there may never have been the United States of America, at least not as we know it today.

- Robert Browne was the man who separated church from state in the reign of Queen Elizabeth 1$^{st}$ which is the underpinning of the United States.
- Robert Browne's words are written into the constitution of the United States.
- Robert Browne's direct descendent officially fired the first shot in the American war of independence.
- Robert Browne's beloved Lilford Hall estate was the home of President George Washington's Mother.
- Robert Browne's beloved Lilford Hall estate was the home of President Quincy Adams' family.

Just like in a horror movie plot, the TV crew of 13 unsuspecting people were thrust into the middle of baffling and extensive paranormal activity.  They experienced doors that refused to stay closed, they had debris thrown at them, they had a door silently ripped away from the hinges and doorframe while they were in the next room.  There were even several recorded multi-witness apparitions of a man fitting Robert Browne's description.  It is believed that the ghost of Robert Browne, the "Grandfather" of the United States as a nation, still haunts Lilford Hall to this day.

### Being American Married to a Brit.

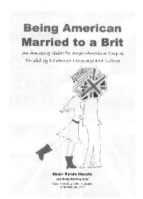

An Amusing Guide for Anglo-American Couples Divided by a Common Language and Culture

When I first started dating my British man, I never gave a second thought about differences in language and culture.  Why would I?  After all, we Americans speak English, or do we…?

As dating quickly turned into being engaged to, and then getting married to my British gentleman, I also found that our common language and culture was a quirky, eye-opening, and highly amusing roller-coaster ride.  At times during the most basic every-day conversations, I'd be listening to his words with glazed eyes, wondering what on earth he was saying.

It really was as if we were both speaking a completely different language, even though the words that

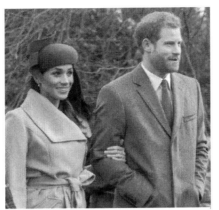

**Meghan Markle and Prince Harry**
Photo by Mark Jones - Wikipedia

comprised the language were the same. I very quickly learned so much more about the language I was supposed to have been taught at school, the commonalities, the differences, and the good old-fashioned belly-laughs about it all that still punctuate our married life to this day. With the Anglo-American Royal Marriage of Prince Harry and Meghan Markle, I decided to write this essential guide and dedicate it to them, and all transatlantic couples who will regularly find themselves completely divided, and confused, by their common language and culture.

www.MajorVision.com

Made in the USA
Middletown, DE
03 December 2018